OPEN-MINDED HEALING

Reclaiming My Health From Autoimmune Disease,
Outside of the MD's Office

MARLA MILLER

Copyright © 2025 Open-Minded Healing, LLC
Marla Miller

www.openmindedhealing.com
Open-Minded Healing: Reclaiming My Health from Autoimmune Disease, Outside of the MD's Office

All rights reserved. No part of this publication may be reproduced, distributed, or transmitted in any form or by any means, including photocopying, recording, or other electronic or mechanical methods, without the prior written permission of the publisher, except in the case of brief quotations embodied in critical reviews and certain other noncommercial uses permitted by copyright law. Neither the author nor the publisher assumes any responsibility or liability whatsoever on behalf of the consumer or reader of this material. Any perceived slight of any individual or organization is purely unintentional. **The resources in this book are provided for informational purposes only and should not be used to replace the specialized training and professional judgement of a health care or mental health care professional.**

Neither the author nor the publisher can be held responsible for the use of the information provided in this book. **Please, always consult a licensed medical professional before making any decision regarding treatment of yourself or others.**

This book is a memoir. It reflects the author's recollections of experiences over time. Some characteristics have been changed, some events have been compressed, some identifying details have been changed, and some dialogue has been recreated. Some names, places, and dates have been changed to protect individual identities and the privacy of their families.

ISBN 979-8-9922287-0-0

Dedication

To my mom and dad — for always encouraging my creativity, curiosity, and spirituality...all of which have contributed to me finding healing.

To my children — for letting me experience the most profound type of love through their existence, and for the great contribution they are making to this world by being their unique selves.

To my cousin, Renee — for being the purest example of love in action, even in the most difficult of times. She suffered greatly from severe health issues but, even up until her death, showed endless love and compassion for those around her.

TABLE OF CONTENTS

Preface ix
Introduction xi

Chapter 1: The Telltale Signs 1
Chapter 2: Thanksgiving Health Woes 5
Chapter 3: A Laundry List of Medications 13
Chapter 4: Healing Groundwork 17
Chapter 5: Heartburn or Heart Attack? 21
Chapter 6: Detoxing Every Aspect 25
Chapter 7: The Power of Meditation 29
Chapter 8: A Pharmacist in the Family 33
Chapter 9: Learn to Speak Up 37
Chapter 10: Become a Super Sleuth 41
Chapter 11: More Much-Needed Family Support 45
Chapter 12: A Heavy Metal Cleanse 47
Chapter 13: Reading Breakthroughs 57
Chapter 14: Releasing What No Longer Serves You 61
Chapter 15: Physical & Spiritual Detoxing 65
Chapter 16: Energetic Shifts 69
Chapter 17: Progress & Setbacks 71
Chapter 18: Adventures & Medical Diaries 73
Chapter 19: A Visit to Ketut Liyer's Home 79
Chapter 20: Thanksgiving Rolls Around Again 85
Chapter 21: Time to Grow a New Body 87
Chapter 22: Holidays & Vivid Dreams 95

Chapter 23: A Costly Journey 99
Chapter 24: From Appointments to Gratitude 103
Chapter 25: Inspiration is All Around You 107
Chapter 26: Gut Health & Tapping 109
Chapter 27: Advocating for the Right Treatments 113
Chapter 28: A Wake-up Call to Go Grain-Free 117
Chapter 29: A Toothy Grin 121
Chapter 30: Taxi Talks & Tucson 125
Chapter 31: Keep Testing 127
Chapter 32: Could It be Toxic Mold? 135
Chapter 33: Healing Strides and Tiny Miracles 137
Chapter 34: Minerals, Nutrients, & Parasites 141
Chapter 35: Major Improvements 145
Chapter 36: Continued Healing & Cleansing 147
Chapter 37: Dentistry Wins 153
Chapter 38: The Future of Self-Healing 155
Chapter 39: Looking Back 157
Chapter 40: Parting Advice 165

Resources: The "How To" Handbook 169
Recommended Reading & Listening 179
References & Citations 181

Acknowledgements

A special thank you to my amazing editor, Madi Miller. Your ability to revise my writing while staying true to the original message I wanted to convey is a true talent. I was blessed to work with you on this project and appreciate your dedication and skill.

I also want to acknowledge all the wonderful health care practitioners and doctors who remained open-minded, listened patiently to my concerns, and embraced my proactive approach to finding healing for myself, all while offering compassionate care along the way.

I will be eternally grateful to my mom, dad, and brother, for taking the time to fly out and help me in whatever ways they could (whether it was taking on tasks I could no longer handle or boosting my morale with their humor and kindness).

I want to acknowledge my friend, Frank, for his continuous emotional support and encouragement as I healed, even as he was struggling with his own health battles. It just goes to show that one person can truly make a profound difference in the life of another. I'm not sure he knows how much of a positive impact he had on me, but maybe he will now.

Thanks go out to the many friends and family members who reached out to lend their support during this time. I will always remember each of you with love and heartfelt appreciation.

I am also grateful for the many strangers I met along the way who didn't hesitate to extend kindness to me. All of you make this world a better, more loving place!

PREFACE

I wrote this book to help anyone out there who is struggling with an autoimmune disease. By sharing the various healing modalities that I've tried and the overall experiences I've had along my path to personal recovery, I hope to help others heal and eliminate unnecessary pain in their own lives while also offering support to anyone who feels lonely, disconnected, or discouraged on their own journey to better health.

Although I'll share a wide array of treatments, some of which I traveled outside the U.S. to explore, it's by no means necessary for you to follow my exact path in order to heal, or to devote the same amount of financial resources as I did in the process. Throughout this book, you'll find plenty of budget-friendly ways to better your health, as well as a general protocol that can prove useful for anyone battling an autoimmune disease.

Keep in mind that no road to recovery looks completely the same. There are many factors that make each person's healing process unique, including varying levels of toxicity, number of years the disease has ravaged their body, capacity to absorb vital nutrients, individual stress levels or trauma, and much more. The information I provide is meant to offer a roadmap to healing from where you currently stand with your health. It's important to avoid comparing your timeline to those of others with the same disease, instead remembering to compare your progress to where you stood a week, a month, or a year before the current moment in time.

It's my sincerest goal to inspire people to take charge of their own health care, trust their instincts, and become their own biggest advocates, both inside and outside of the doctor's office. Even when the road ahead seems uncertain, trust that your efforts — big or small, common or unconventional — will make a difference in how you feel.

If my story resonates with you, inspires you, educates you, offers you hope, or ultimately leads you on your own road to recovery, this book will have served its purpose.

Introduction

It has been my mission, for the longest time, to share my story so that others may find solutions for putting their own autoimmune diseases into remission and harness hope for a symptom-free future. Although I am not a licensed medical professional, I've experienced the diagnosis of an autoimmune condition firsthand, as well as the recovery made possible by my pursuit of unconventional healing modalities. I pursued these alternative avenues in order to heal my body physically, emotionally, and spiritually. I would like to share my experiences with you so that you might find the insights you need to kickstart your personal path to recovery. The information shared here is based on personal experience and should not be considered medical advice.

One thing I want everyone to take away from all of this is the fact that there is hope for healing and that you are not alone in this process.

Understanding the Long Road Ahead

There is no simple solution to a complicated disease. Recovery is a process that will require patience as you heal one layer at a time. I believe it's important to remember that the disease you're suffering from started long before your symptoms surfaced. For some of you, your own path to symptomatic disease may have been 20 to 30 years in the making. Understanding how long it took to bring your body to this precipice should tell you that your healing — or undoing — processes will take time as well.

Each day throughout your healing journey, ask yourself if you're moving forward — even if it's one small step at a time. I highly recommend taking detailed notes of your daily actions in a special journal to monitor your progress. This is exactly what I did, and it is from these notes that I have based this book. If you can do this, you'll be able to remind yourself just how far you have come.

Even if nobody has been in your corner up until this point, know this: **I'm rooting for you!**

The Power of Your Beliefs

Before you dive into this book, I need to address the power of your beliefs. I use the word "believe" frequently because I think it carries significant weight, especially when you are trying to heal yourself. Your beliefs have the power to determine whether or not you'll have a positive health outcome further on in your healing journey.

So, here's what I **believe**. If you truly believe that you will get better, that sense of conviction can have a majorly positive impact on your recovery. On the opposite side of that coin, your lack of belief can be just as detrimental to your health. If you think there's no hope for overcoming your condition, your body and your mind will remain stuck. If you believe a medical doctor holds all the answers to your recovery, it may stop you from finding other real solutions. Whether you believe the Universe is conspiring on your behalf or against you will completely change the outcome of your day, along with the state of your health.

I'll give you a prime example of the word "belief" in action. One day, when I was hobbling through Whole Foods on my crutches, a considerate woman offered to let me put my groceries in her basket as I shopped. Our conversation veered toward the topic of health, and it turned out that she had also been diagnosed with an autoimmune condition. She seemed worn out and disheartened, expressing that she had already gone through a few surgeries as a result of her disease. I shared my personal diagnosis, telling her that I was not having it — this disease — and that this was not my life. I would not **let** this be my life. I said this with a small smile but meant it quite seriously. She seemed a little shocked by that statement and responded, "But you **do** have it." I wasn't going to argue my point to a woman who had clearly been through a lot of pain battling a debilitating disease, but in my own mind I was saying, "Yes, I do have it, but not for long."

I have never identified with this diagnosis. It is something that I live with, not a part of who I am. I don't know if this mindset stemmed from an innate understanding that this illness didn't belong to me for the long term or a delusionally optimistic determination to heal at all costs. Some might say that perhaps I was in denial. One thing I do know for sure is that my unwavering belief that this illness was not mine to keep was one key to my recovery.

I think each individual holds the real power in healing. You must have hope that you will find solutions for recovering your health and you must **believe** that you will get better. What you focus on expands, so if you're continuously focusing on dire outcomes, a lack of finances or resources, or a victim mentality, the resonance of those thoughts will unwittingly invite more of the same into your life. On the other hand, if you remain optimistic and open-minded, you'll be more attuned to the potential solutions put in front of you.

Determine precisely what you need, and then communicate it clearly to the Universe without including all the things that you lack or don't want.

Whether you believe in a higher power of some sort or not, your belief in a better future for yourself will determine just how far you'll go on your healing journey. Now I would like to invite you to take a front-row seat to my healing journey. I hope that these stories, and the practical advice therein, will inspire you to take a proactive approach in your own life.

CHAPTER 1

The Telltale Signs

I've always wanted to start a book off with *"It was a dark and stormy night..."* but that wouldn't be true in this case.

It was actually a very bright and balmy day in September 2015 when I arrived at my friend Kate's house in sunny San Diego, California. I was visiting for a few days from San Jose and planned on taking some modeling photos of her daughter, Lisa, while I was there.

Later that day, we had settled in with a delicious dinner and some great conversation when my right foot became noticeably swollen and uncomfortable. I guessed, at the time, that it was probably due to sitting for so long during my eight-hour drive earlier that day. I proceeded to ice my foot and pop some extra-strength Advil, brushing it off as a temporary side effect of my travels. The following day, however, the swelling persisted, and it was becoming incredibly uncomfortable. We decided to continue with the photo shoot at the beach, even though it was getting increasingly difficult to ignore the pain in my foot as I struggled to walk across the sand.

That trip went by in a blur of pain, and as soon as I got back to San Jose, I booked an appointment with my family physician, who ordered blood work and scheduled X-rays to determine if there was a fracture in my foot. There was not. He ruled out gout and diabetes through the blood work but informed me that I was extremely anemic — red flag number one!

The doctor was quite surprised that this condition had not been discovered prior to our appointment since the storage of iron in my system was almost completely depleted. The blood panel showed that my ferritin level was at 4 ng/mL when it should have been in the range of 13–150 ng/mL, according to Mount Sinai Hospital. This would explain the sheer exhaustion I had been experiencing over the previous few months that had resigned me to taking a nap each day without fail. One day I had even slept all the way through until 4 p.m.

Even though I had spent the past summer eating spinach salads daily, along with other foods rich in iron, my body didn't seem to be breaking down and absorbing the nutrients properly. The doctor put me on a daily dose of liquid iron for better absorption and suggested that I follow up with a podiatrist.

The podiatrist ordered additional X-rays which, again, didn't show anything conclusive. He suggested that I try on an orthopedic boot to see if it would take the pressure off my foot and allow me to walk around without limping. There was no way I could push my swollen foot into a compressed boot without serious discomfort, so I took a hard pass on that idea. I even tried to escape his office while he was consulting with another patient after he mentioned the prospect of a needle biopsy procedure. For those of you who don't know what this is, it's a procedure that would require fluid to be drawn from my swollen foot with a needle to gain more conclusive information. After the doctor caught me in my attempted disappearing act, I explained that I couldn't let anyone put even slight pressure on my foot, let alone stick a needle into it!

We agreed that I could forgo the biopsy and set up an appointment with a rheumatologist instead. I left his office with a sense of relief from having escaped the needle but with the fast-growing fear of still not having the answers I had hoped to find.

Earlier in the month, I had blood work done through my naturopath. I went to her office to obtain the results and found that I was low in vitamin C, manganese, copper, and B vitamins. This explained why my iron levels were so low: I lacked all the nutrients and minerals necessary for absorbing iron. The synergistic relationship of various nutrients is complex, which is why it's so important for vitamins and minerals to be balanced in your body. Each one plays a key role in how the other nutrients function and, ultimately, how your body functions as a whole.

My neurotransmitter testing showed that I had reached stage 3 adrenal fatigue and that my cortisol was incredibly low. My adrenal glands had become so stressed that they were incapable of producing a healthy amount of cortisol. This would explain why I had been struggling to wake up and stay awake throughout the day and perhaps why my immune system wasn't performing optimally.

"When you're stressed, your adrenal glands, which sit atop the kidneys, produce a hormone called cortisol. Cortisol helps your body respond effectively to stress. It also plays a role in bone health, immune system response, and the metabolism of food." [1]

It's important to note that any source of chronic stress can have a major physiological impact on our health, sometimes even serving as a trigger for autoimmune disease. In order to get a complete picture of your health, it's crucial to know how your body is functioning on all levels. I recommend working with a naturopath, functional medicine doctor, or similar health care professional to conduct tests that will be more comprehensive than the ones an MD might typically order.

*

There are always telltale signs of poor health that often go ignored. In the coming chapter, you'll see how I began to piece the puzzle together.

CHAPTER 2

THANKSGIVING HEALTH WOES

"The most fertile source of insight is hindsight."
~Morris Kline

By Thanksgiving, my foot had become unbearable to walk on, and it had become necessary to purchase crutches. My foot was so swollen that my toes were actually stuck together, and I needed to elevate and ice my foot regularly. I couldn't even put a sock on my foot anymore because it had become so swollen and uncomfortable. I wouldn't allow anyone to come within a *foot* of my foot, in fear that they would bump into it.

The rheumatologist wanted to take X-rays, but I put my foot down — the good one, that is — and explained that I didn't want any excess radiation affecting my body if it wasn't necessary. This was one of many times that I would be insistent about my own care. **Many times, doctors will suggest certain courses of action because they have a particular order of protocol, not because it's completely necessary.**

The doctor offered an MRI as an alternative, which would give us a little more information without exposing me to the harmful radiation from the X-ray. After leaving her office, I went home and anxiously awaited the results.

The Diagnosis

It was the very beginning of December 2015 when I received the call from the rheumatologist asking me to come to her office. She was reluctant to give me the results of my MRI over the phone, which raised instant alarm bells. Upon arriving at the office, I tried to quell my nerves as I waited impatiently for my name to be called. Once we were in private, the doctor broke the news quite casually, informing me that I had rheumatoid arthritis. I burst into tears.

I knew enough about this disease to understand the crippling effects that it can have on the body. My mind jumped to the worst-case scenario, envisioning a life full of terrible pain. At that moment, the doctor mentioned that, although there was no cure, I could still lead a productive life. Her words rang hollow, deafened by my own dark thoughts. I genuinely believed that my life was over, convinced that my low threshold for pain would make this condition unbearable.

The doctor immediately scribbled down a prescription for prednisone as well as methotrexate, a drug commonly used to treat autoimmune conditions. She also suggested getting a cortisone shot in my foot. It felt like she was throwing everything in her arsenal my way in order to feel like she had done her job. Whether everything she prescribed was warranted or not was yet to be seen. I declined the offer of cortisone, as I didn't desire the pain of a shot in my swollen foot or the addition of a medication that may or may not have benefited me in the long run. My first dosage of methotrexate was taken on December 5, along with the prednisone. I would normally never consider taking either of these medications because of the harmful side effects and overall toll they take on your body, but when the doctor stated that the medication would take a few months to start working (while my bones would continue to deteriorate in the meantime), I relented. I convinced myself that the medication would only be a temporary fix — just until I could come up with my own cure.

There Is No Cure

Whenever I hear the words "there is no cure" from a doctor, it just means that the doctor is not aware of a cure at that moment in time. I believe that it's possible to find a cure for every affliction in the world. However, if we close our minds to other possible solutions and keep adhering to the same protocols that merely mask our symptoms, rather than healing the underlying cause, we will remain stuck in a state of disease.

We need to delve deeper into finding the root cause of our issues. From there, we can work toward a complete remission or cure. By keeping an open mind and exploring healing modalities from an array of different cultures, we can find solutions. In my opinion, if your doctor is adamant that there's nothing they can do but put you on medication for the rest of your life, you need to keep searching for another doctor — as well as other remedies.

In the initial stages of my diagnosis, I searched for others who had healed from rheumatoid arthritis. Although my search didn't produce many promising results, I did find a book by Henry Scammell and Thomas McPherson Brown titled *The Road Back: Rheumatoid Arthritis — Its Cause and Its Treatment*. I devoured all of the information provided by the authors, which served as a great starting point for me because it gave me hope that I would find a cure. It also inspired me to cultivate a deeper understanding of the causes of rheumatoid arthritis.

"What is called the autoimmune reaction in all these forms of arthritis is actually the body's natural defense against an infection in the connective tissues. The body attacks disease agents that cling to the cells or are embedded within them." (2)

As I continued my quest for knowledge about the disease, I discovered the theory that mycoplasmas cause rheumatoid arthritis, and that these mycoplasmas can be treated with tetracycline. This spurred me into action. On my next visit to the rheumatologist, I mentioned that I wanted to be tested for mycoplasmas, even though they can escape detection by hiding in your tissues and therefore produce a false negative test result. The doctor said that she didn't believe I had mycoplasmas but went ahead and ordered the test when she saw my determination. The test came back negative.

Environmental Factors

Sometimes, environmental factors can have a big impact on our health. Among the very detailed information offered in *The Road Back* was the mention of the fact that some people with the disease have fared well in warm and dry environments like Phoenix, Arizona. A particular chapter focused on how the barometric pressure in this region remains fairly even throughout the year, which may be helpful because joint pain and stiffness seem to fluctuate along with barometric pressure. I kept this theory in mind and considered spending a month at my parents' house in Tucson to test it out for myself. I also recalled that, years ago, my aunt had suffered from rheumatoid arthritis and was headed toward a life confined to a wheelchair when her doctor recommended that she move from Kansas to Arizona in order to escape more dire days ahead. My aunt took her doctor's advice and moved to Phoenix with her husband. Between frequent swims and daily life in the desert climate, she ultimately ended up going into remission.

Hindsight Is 20/20

The Road Back also mentioned that the first sign of rheumatoid arthritis is actually fatigue, followed by depression and anemia. Contrary to popular belief, pain is not the first indicator. The authors mentioned that many doctors will make the patient feel that they may be responsible for their own condition by leading a stressful life, sometimes even questioning whether the patient is actually adhering to the prescribed protocol when their iron stores don't improve. As a result, the patient goes home without insisting on more tests or answers, defeated by the idea that their sickness is their own doing.

As I looked back on my life, I realized that my current symptoms weren't the first signs of my autoimmune condition. I had experienced consistent stomach issues since a young age but came to accept them as normal. Back in grade school, I never brought a traditional lunch of peanut butter & jelly sandwiches and milk to school since I wasn't a fan of milk or bread. Come to think of it, maybe my body knew something I was yet to discover regarding gluten and dairy. Throughout high school, my stomach was always overly sensitive, and I frequently struggled with serious bloating and sharp pains that left me wanting to skip school altogether — although my mom never let that fly.

Later, when my own children were little, I went to the doctor because my knees had become visibly swollen, making it painful to walk. Testing showed that I had a minor case of rheumatoid arthritis. As it was so minor, the doctor didn't mention doing anything to remedy it at that time. This appointment took place during a particularly stressful period in my life when we were determining whether uprooting our family from the East Coast to the West Coast was the right choice. During that same time period, I was also getting migraine headaches that eventually drove me to see a neurologist, who insisted it was nothing to worry about and suggested I see a dentist for a possible temporomandibular joint (TMJ) issue. After making the official move to California, the knee pain persisted for about six more months. Then, one day, it went away on its own, so I didn't give it any more thought.

Several years later, when my children were both in grade school, I was experiencing issues with my stomach on a regular basis, so I went to see the family doctor. No tests were ever run, and the doctor chalked it up to irritable bowel syndrome (IBS) without offering any solutions. The following year, I would go back to the same doctor with complaints of exhaustion, which he would attribute to the stress of being a mom to two small children.

My total reliance on MDs and their conventional protocols came to an end right after a family reunion in Oregon. My ears had become watery and quite itchy, and I initially assumed it was from the time I had spent swimming in the lake during the trip. The doctor checked my ears and said he didn't see anything out of the ordinary but prescribed an antibiotic based on my self-described symptoms. I decided not to take the antibiotic, considering that I hadn't even received a diagnosis. That was the day I decided to start seeing a naturopath in hopes that she could get to the root cause of my fatigue and itchy ears.

At my first appointment, the naturopath put a scope into my ears and immediately confirmed eczema as the culprit. This made sense to me since I remembered having painful eczema on my hands when I was in my 20s. The symptoms were the same and it did run in my family, but I was surprised to discover that this particular condition could affect your ears as well. After running another panel of tests, including food allergy and nutrient deficiency testing, she was able to confirm a host of other gut-health-related issues as well as an MTHFR gene mutation, both of which I'll elaborate on later in this book.

This was the day that the naturopath became my primary care doctor.

Exercise: Uncovering the Unexplained

I'd like you to do a bit of an exercise at this point. I want you to try to track all your health conditions and illnesses that were either unexplainable or treated without a conclusive diagnosis. These collective little clues might very well help solidify a diagnosis or direct you to the right treatment. Using a journal, take a moment to list your past conditions.

CHAPTER 3

A Laundry List of Medications

"We must be willing to let go of the life we have planned so as to have the life that is waiting for us."

~Joseph Campbell

In January of 2016, I was switching health insurance companies, so I needed to schedule an appointment with a new rheumatologist. This particular rheumatologist encouraged me to take the biologic drug, Humira, to battle the disease. She said it could be taken alongside the prednisone as a replacement for the methotrexate if the methotrexate alone wasn't producing noticeable results. However, that was the last thing I wanted to do. I was trying to get off all medication, not add to the list!

I explained to her that I wouldn't be adding any additional medications and that I planned on weaning off the prednisone right away. My previous doctor had told me that prednisone typically begins working quickly, often providing patients with noticeable relief from inflammation in a matter of days, but I hadn't noticed any difference in my condition since I started it over a month ago.

Although she instructed me to continue taking prednisone as long as any swelling was still present, I wasn't on board. I had already witnessed the devastation that this detrimental drug can wreak on your health by seeing the effects it has had on my brother throughout his years-long battle with Crohn's disease. Prednisone can create a thinning of the bones, deterioration of the teeth, irritation of the gut lining and intestines, mood changes, depression, changes in vision, and a general weakening of the immune system. It's confounding to me that some doctors are so quick to keep a patient on a standard protocol without proof of its effectiveness for that particular individual.

After insisting that I wasn't willing to continue taking a toxic drug that wasn't even helping to relieve any of my symptoms, she agreed to provide me with a plan to wean off it slowly. Although I was initially tempted to quit cold turkey, I was more agreeable to decreasing my dosage gradually once I did some more research on the topic.

NOTE: When you're taking prednisone, it acts similarly to cortisol, so your adrenal glands decrease the production of cortisol. If you decrease your dosage slowly, you can prevent withdrawal symptoms and allow your adrenal glands adequate time to resume their normal functioning.

As I pulled out of the doctor's parking lot, I glanced in the rearview mirror and was frightened by what I saw reflected back. All my teeth seemed to have a black tinge to them. Were my teeth all dying now because of this disease, or did I have a second health issue to worry about? I called my dentist right away, and he was luckily able to squeeze me into his tight schedule that day. Once he saw my teeth, he concluded that the black tint must have originated from something I was eating. I couldn't think of anything that would have had this effect on my teeth until I got home and it suddenly hit me: the liquid iron! I looked up the side effects of liquid iron and found one article that mentioned it may leave a black stain. I wondered why no one had mentioned this to me when I first started taking it but was ultimately relieved that this was the only cause of my black-stained teeth. Only a professional dental cleaning could remove the stains. Since I wasn't about to start making daily trips to the dentist for this purpose, I decided that I would just live with it until I was done with the liquid iron completely and could get my teeth professionally cleaned. While there were occasional moments when I'd be reminded of my "tainted beauty" by an appalled look on someone's face as we chatted, it didn't bother me much since my lack of mobility typically kept my socializing to a minimum.

Getting Another Opinion

I decided to see one more rheumatologist, who I'll call "Dr. S.", who had been recommended by a close friend. My friend insisted that he was well-educated and open to other modes of healing in addition to the drugs typically prescribed for arthritis. Thanks to the insights I had picked up from *The Road Back*, I was able to write down a list of informed questions for Dr. S before my appointment. I mentioned what I had previously read about mycoplasmas being the cause of arthritis and how my test had come back negative. I went on to add that I wondered if he could treat my condition with tetracycline, just in case it had been a false negative.

I'm normally not one for adding in medications that might worsen my condition, but all signs pointed to tetracycline being more healing than harmful. Dr. S patiently answered all my questions but ultimately advised against it, assuring me that it wouldn't be beneficial in my case. He also emphasized that proper diet, sleep, and stress management were key components of healing. After carefully reviewing my symptoms, medical records, and family history, he amended my initial diagnosis of rheumatoid arthritis to ankylosing spondylitis, another chronic progressive inflammatory disease. He took note of the fact that both my brother and my niece have Crohn's disease, an autoimmune condition stemming from the gut. Additionally, my sister has alopecia, an autoimmune condition that has caused her to lose all of her hair. There definitely seemed to be a genetic factor at play.

I decided to keep the diagnosis to myself for the time being. I didn't want people looking up this disease and associating it with me, and I didn't want to envision anything other than perfect health for myself. Despite the fact that Dr. S was out of network and his consultations came at a cost, I decided to continue working with him because I trusted him the most out of the three rheumatologists I had seen. Paying out of pocket seemed like a small price to pay for the promise of a healthy future. He even agreed to work in conjunction with my other rheumatologist, happily forwarding any results and recommended tests so that she could stay in the loop.

I can't tell you how important it is to find a doctor who is willing to work with you; one that wants to do more than just fill out a prescription and send you on your way so they can move on to the next patient in their queue.

Exercise: Medical History Mapping

In the exercise from the previous chapter, you created a list of your prior health conditions. Now, if you can, I would like you to do some medical history tracing with your family members. Your parents, siblings, and siblings' children might have symptoms of illnesses that can help you learn more about your own condition. Use your journal to create this list once you've reached out to your family members.

CHAPTER 4

HEALING GROUNDWORK

"Sometimes when you're in a dark place, you think you've been buried, but you've actually been planted."
~Christine Caine

Following the initial news that I had a condition that was associated with a lot of pain and multiple surgeries — one that had no cure — I spiraled into a state of depression. After several days of what my mom would call a "pity party," I decided to start thinking of solutions rather than problems. I read up on autoimmune diseases and learned that certain ones are related to the health of your gut. In my search for more answers, I came across Dr. Josh Axe and his crusade for healing a condition known as leaky gut. Dr. Axe seemed so well-informed that I decided to purchase a membership to his online program, which included a wealth of helpful information about healing the gut as well as access to a support group on Facebook.

After joining the program, I jumped wholeheartedly into a drastic diet change. For the next three months, I eliminated dairy, gluten, and grains. I also did away with corn, soy, sugar, and pork. I was now on crutches full-time, finding it extremely difficult to get around. On top of that, I was physically exhausted and could barely get anything accomplished at home, let alone make the effort to leave the house. As a result, I was able to eliminate all food in my pantry and refrigerator that wasn't a part of my new diet, thus avoiding temptation. When I say that I eliminated sugar, I mean that I had ZERO sugar, including the natural sugars found in fruit. My fear of pain was greater than my addiction to sugar! Who knew?

My condition, as well as the new diet, left me feeling completely drained and quite hungry. I found myself needing to rest for most of the day and sit with my foot propped up on a nearby table with an ice pack applied. I was basically existing on certified organic chicken and ground turkey, lots of organic vegetables, coconut aminos (for flavoring), and all-organic bone broth soup.

Moving forward, my life seemed to be centered around the kitchen — a place I preferred to avoid in favor of takeout before falling ill — and preparing my next meal in advance. I had to rely on friends and family for lots of support, including grocery store runs and some meal prep. Because of my lack of mobility, I gravitated toward online shopping at this time, browsing for groceries, books on health and spirituality, and various healing products from the comfort of my couch. This not only saved me the strenuous effort of leaving the house but brought me some much-needed moments of joy that came in the form of new packages on my front porch.

Daily Difficulties

I didn't realize just how difficult it would be to accomplish everyday tasks on crutches until I experienced it for myself. There were some things, like taking out the garbage, that became impossible for me to do since they required two free hands. Going down any set of steps became a daily challenge, and there were many times I nearly missed and fell flat on the pavement as I tried to balance my body weight against the pull of gravity. Taking a shower was a feat in itself since I couldn't put any weight on my right foot. My son offered to come home if I needed his help, even though he was living a few hours away at the time. My daughter was away at college but was extremely helpful when she returned home for her three-week Christmas break. She took care of the laundry, kept my ice pack filled, ran to the store, and made sure I was all settled in my bed at night before she went to sleep. I must admit that initially, when my children were home for the holidays, they still expected me to operate at the same capacity as I had before my diagnosis and newfound dependency on crutches. It took me breaking down in tears one night for them to understand the severity of my condition and the serious toll it was taking on me. After an emotional conversation and many appreciated hugs, they were both fully on board with lending me assistance. Why am I telling you this? Because you shouldn't be afraid to let people know exactly how you're feeling or to explicitly ask for their help.

Of course, there are many tangible solutions to autoimmune diseases, which we will continue exploring, but **love** should not be overlooked as a healing agent. Knowing that I was surrounded by people who loved me and were willing to go so far out of their way to help truly contributed to my positive health outcome.

Exercise: Assembling Your Support Team

Even if you've told your family and friends about your autoimmune condition, they still may not fully understand the many ways that it will impact your life. If you can, try to call a meeting with your immediate family and express the level of support that you hope to have from them. Sometimes, people want to help but simply don't know how. Using your journal, write down specific tasks you would love to have assistance with, then share it with the people who are willing to help.

Communication is key when you're living with a condition like this.

CHAPTER 5

Heartburn or Heart Attack?

On one of my daughter's last nights at home before her return to school, I was woken up suddenly in the middle of the night by a tight sensation in my chest. I thought that it might be heartburn and waited to see if it would go away. The feeling gradually worsened until it felt like there was a tight vice around my chest. After calling out to my daughter from down the hall, she came into the room and saw my panicked state. I asked her to Google symptoms of a heart attack, but I knew if I was actually having one, we were wasting valuable time. I quickly dialed 911. By the time the Fire Department arrived, my daughter was waiting at the front door to let in the five robust young men who were all geared up and ready to avert tragedy. They made their way to my bedroom at the back of the house, which was looking quite cluttered. You see, by this point in my healing journey, I had developed the habit of leaving all my clothes on the bed to make it more convenient to dress in the morning on crutches. I think they were a bit taken aback by my disheveled appearance. My hair was messy, my teeth were stained black from the liquid iron, and I had dark circles under my eyes. I was momentarily distracted from my own possible heart attack as I contemplated how my current appearance may have induced a heart attack in one of my rescuers. As one fireman approached, I was pounding my chest, thinking that I would either dislodge whatever was causing my indigestion or pump my malfunctioning heart back into action. He seemed irritated with me as he asked me to stop pounding my chest. The same fireman asked me to take two chewable aspirin, to which I responded, "Do I chew them?" His terse response of, "That's why I said chewable," let me know that I had exasperated him further. I think his irritation came from the fact that I was questioning everything he was asking me to do. Although he may have thought I was trying to give him a hard time, I was simply not thinking clearly that night. They gave me something to put under my tongue, then measured my vitals while we waited for the ambulance. They also asked my daughter if I suffered from anxiety. While I typically have a consistently calm demeanor, this night was definitely far from typical. The paramedics finally came to my rescue and transported me to the hospital. On the way, one of them asked me why I was so anxious. I explained that I had just recently been diagnosed with an autoimmune condition and now the thought that I may be having a heart attack was putting me over the edge, especially since I had never been seriously ill prior to my recent diagnosis.

After many tests and hours spent at the hospital, I was released with a diagnosis of gastroesophageal reflux disease (GERD). I believe that it was triggered by the bison burger that I had eaten shortly before bedtime the previous night (which was almost worth the ambulance ride). The hospital sent me home with an antacid, but I already knew based on past testing that what I really needed was more digestive enzymes, not something that was going to dilute the limited acid in my stomach. I decided not to take the antacid the hospital had prescribed and, instead, took one Rhizinate 3X: a natural digestive treatment that was given to me by the naturopath, which I would take on the rare occasions when I was experiencing heartburn. Going forward, I never experienced anything like that night again; something I credit to my trusty digestive enzymes (taken with each meal) and my determination to curb any late-night snacking.

The Benefits of Digestive Enzymes

Most digestive enzymes are made by the pancreas. If your pancreas can't make these enzymes sufficiently, it can make digestion a terrible ordeal. If you have symptoms of reflux, silent reflux (laryngopharyngeal reflux), or gastroesophageal reflux disease, it's important to investigate natural remedies that can aid in digestion and help balance your gut enzymes. Symptoms can include:

- Chest pains and a burning sensation in your chest
- Difficulty swallowing
- Regurgitation of food or sour liquids
- Globus sensation (persistent feeling of a lump in your throat that doesn't go away when you swallow)

Be aware that if you are an inherently anxious person, this can trigger acid production in your stomach and lead to a weakening in the esophageal sphincters that work to close your stomach off from your esophageal tube. Now, for some people with silent reflux, the only symptoms they have are pain and a globus sensation in the throat, along with a hoarse voice. This can be incredibly unsettling because the symptoms can crop up out of nowhere. Taking care of your gut health with the aid of digestive enzymes won't just help with your reflux but with your overall health too!

CHAPTER 6

Detoxing Every Aspect

"A mind is like a parachute. It doesn't work if it isn't open."
~Frank Zappa

In my search for healing, I came upon a series of detoxing solutions for the home and began implementing various ideas. I bought filters for both of my showerheads to eliminate chlorine and other toxins, as well as an air filter to remove allergens and potential pollutants from my bedroom. I also purchased a special hard-bristled brush for dry brushing my skin. For those of you who aren't aware of what dry brushing is, it's a form of body massage that aids circulation and lymphatic drainage while exfoliating your skin.

After researching infrared saunas, I found that they are fantastic for detoxing the body and offer many other healing benefits as well. I decided to buy an infrared healing mat as a compromise — much less expensive than a home sauna but still effective! I got rid of all of my Teflon-coated pans to eliminate the possibility of heavy metals seeping into my food from the cookware, joking to myself that this was just another welcomed sign to abandon cooking altogether. I also purchased a high-quality countertop water filter to protect my body from absorbing chlorine and other harmful contaminants.

Getting into a Routine

After some trial and error, I developed a routine that seemed to work for me. During the daytime, I would lie on the infrared mat and meditate for 30 minutes. The heat, as well as the detoxifying effects, made me noticeably tired but also released any immediate pain I was feeling. Each night, I would get settled in bed by 8 p.m. and place an ice pack on my foot before it became too uncomfortable, playing the therapeutic music of <u>Wholetones</u> and the meditation CD by Esther Hicks, *"Getting into the Vortex,"* as I fell asleep. This nightly ritual provided me with comfort and much-needed sleep. If you haven't heard of *Wholetones: The Healing Frequency Music Project* by Michael S. Tyrrell, I would suggest checking it out in the Recommended Reading & Listening section at the end of this book.

At the end of February, I called my mom and mentioned that I had been experiencing a foreign feeling. It was so strange. For about six weeks, I had been filled with so much love and positivity. Everywhere I went, I couldn't help but start a conversation with each person I walked past, never having to search too hard for the best qualities in every stranger on the street. I also found that I was in a fantastic mood every day and that nothing could subdue my high spirits. This spoke volumes since I had been feeling somewhat depressed for several months up until that point.

Another unusual occurrence during this six-week period was my heightened awareness of any surrounding negativity. I avoided anything even remotely negative during this timeframe, including the news and negative talk. When people would speak, I would pick up on anything that was even slightly cynical, which, in the past, I would have considered nothing more than normal conversation.

I joked with my mom that maybe this new and improved mood of mine was a result of my gluten-free lifestyle. However, I later ruled this out because while my diet would remain consistent, that mood would not. Possibly it was the elimination of all sugar during those six weeks, although I don't know how that would correlate to my newfound aversion to any form of negativity. I guess we can all choose to believe what we want, but I choose to believe that the extreme love that I felt in those weeks was a direct result of divine intervention. Thanks to my consistent deep meditation practice, transparent requests for assistance, elevated mindset, and truly nourishing diet, I believed I had raised my frequency to a high enough level that Divine Beings were letting me *feel* their presence! Or perhaps I had just let go of all resistance and was now open to the infinite, ever-present Divine Energy of Love — something we ALL encompass at our core.

Exercise: Signs from the Universe

If you're looking for reassurance that the Universe is constantly conspiring on your behalf, you'll find it in life's subtle synchronicities — meaningful coincidences that seem related or connected in a way that goes beyond mere chance. These events serve as signs that you are in the "flow" and on the right path.

The following is a brief list of possible synchronicities that you might be overlooking in your own life. In your journal, jot down all the synchronicities you experience.

- The same number(s) appearing wherever you go
- An unexpected call from an old friend when they randomly cross your mind
- Relevant answers or solutions flowing freely into your life
- Randomly meeting people who offer helpful pieces to your personal health puzzle

CHAPTER 7

THE POWER OF MEDITATION

"You cannot find the solution to any problem when the problem is the most active Vibration within you."

~Abraham Hicks

Why do I believe it's so important to incorporate meditation into your journey toward self-healing?

I personally find it to be a phenomenal way to reduce stress and manifest the healthy life you desire. I know it can be difficult for some people to get into initially, but it's so worthwhile to establish this healing habit. Initially, I would get distracted easily or fall asleep. However, as I persisted and developed a routine — meditating daily in the same serene space I had created for myself — I became more entranced each time. If I became stressed out during the day with finances or health issues, I would feel the immediate urge to meditate because I knew how great it would make me feel. In the moments when anxiety would start to rule, I was quick to banish it with a short meditation session, feeling calm, clear-headed, and confident I could find solutions to any perceived problems upon opening my eyes.

What I've learned is that two different parts of the brain control your creative problem-solving capacity (the prefrontal cortex) and your fight-or-flight response (the amygdala). You cannot access these two parts of the brain simultaneously. When you're in stress mode, the amygdala — at the base of your brain — takes control. When you're relaxed, you can access the decision-making portion of your brain, known as the prefrontal cortex, at the front of your brain. Moving from your hindbrain to your front brain is an important step to calming down and conquering daily challenges. Ultimately, if you're stuck in an anxious state, it can prevent you from finding helpful solutions to the problems life throws your way. The best way I've found to disengage the fight-or-flight response is to quiet the mind through a meditative state.

The Key to Meditation

The key to meditation is not only envisioning what general outcome you hope to achieve but also actually feeling the emotion of obtaining your dreams while you meditate. If you feel the excitement in your body, as if you've already attained what you're seeking, your body will respond as if it has happened. Ultimately, this puts you in that higher vibrational state that attracts what you want.

I'd like to leave you with an excerpt on the matter from The Tremendous Power of Meditation by Nayaswami Jyotish:

"When the body is completely relaxed, the five senses become stilled, and the mind becomes deeply focused; a tremendous flow of energy becomes available. That intense energy can lift us into superconsciousness, where our inner powers of intuition are fully awakened. Deep meditation helps us become aware of realities barely dreamed of. And even a little internalization of our consciousness lifts us toward that state and brings great peace. Physiologically, meditation has been found to reduce stress, strengthen the immune system, and help regulate many of the body's systems. During meditation, the breath slows, blood pressure and metabolic rates decrease, and circulation and detoxification of the blood increase." (3)

Exercise: *Mindfulness Meditation*

This mindfulness meditation exercise is an easy introduction to meditation. It's a simple practice that you can use every day to slow your mind down and become more conscious of your actions. Sadly, when we're diagnosed with diseases of this nature, the anxiety and trauma of the discovery can inadvertently sink us deeper into a non-conscious, autopilot frame of mind. As such, using mindfulness will help you find your true north again so that you can focus on healing. To get started:

1. Start by playing one of the videos below.
2. Adopt an attitude of gratitude.
3. Listen to and/or say the chants along with the video.
4. Ask or tell the Universe what you want or how to achieve it yourself, only using positive terms. (For example, reframe the statement, "I don't want to be sick," as "I want to be healthy.")
5. Spend some time with the chants, saying them aloud or in your mind.
6. Remain silent with the meditation for as long as you can or want.

Morning Meditation ("Ah" Chants)
https://youtu.be/046ezMfvZs8

Evening Meditation ("Om" Chants)
https://youtu.be/LMmuChXra_M

Practice these meditations for 90 days to achieve your desired goal or be shown the path to getting it.

You are the co-creator of this Universe. By aligning your mindset and your energy, you can create the reality you most desire.

CHAPTER 8

A Pharmacist in the Family

"Most of all, differences of opinion are opportunities for learning."
~Terry Tempest Williams

After my daughter's Christmas visit came to an end, I realized that I would soon need additional assistance. I called my parents, confiding that I couldn't get by on my own at this time and really needed their help. Even though they weren't around to see the seriousness of my situation firsthand, they knew that I wouldn't be calling them with this request unless it was truly important.

My parents took turns flying out to spend a week with me, as did my brother. They were a tremendous source of love and support. Between my family and friends, I was able to receive much-needed help with grocery shopping, cleaning, walking my dog, preparing meals, and completing various other tasks around the house.

My dad was the first to arrive. As a real go-getter who doesn't sit idle for long, he was eager to run errands for me and take my dog, Lucy, for a walk each day. He also accompanied me to my various doctor's appointments and encouraged me to get a knee scooter to have more mobility than I had with the crutches. The knee scooter turned out to be a fantastic idea (chalk one up for dad)! Now I could zoom around the kitchen and use both hands to prepare meals.

While my dad was visiting, he noticed the many supplements I was taking and expressed his concern at the fact that an MD had not prescribed them. He had worked for a pharmaceutical company throughout his entire career and was quite convinced that conventional medicine was the only way to go. I explained to him that I had been willing to hear the MDs out — and had been taking the medications they had prescribed — but that they weren't actually offering me a cure for my condition. The supplements I was taking alongside the medications were given to me by my naturopath following the results of the blood draws, urine tests, and stool tests that determined that my body needed them to heal. I added some additional supplements based on my own research, such as krill oil with astaxanthin, to mitigate the effects of prednisone on my eyesight.

NOTE: Prednisone can cause blurred vision, sudden headaches, and other changes in vision.

Although fish oil and krill oil both provide beneficial omega-3 fatty acids (DHA and EPA), research shows that krill oil is more easily absorbed and contains the naturally occurring antioxidant astaxanthin.

I further explained to my dad that the prescribed medications had serious side effects, and I refused to be on them for life as the doctors had suggested. As a result, I had made a conscious decision to test other methods of healing until I was completely free of all of my symptoms and had put this disease into remission or found a complete cure.

My dad asked why I was getting so worked up in my response, and I realized that he was just asking questions out of love and concern for my well-being. I wasn't actually upset with him. I had just become passionate about the topic because there are so many people out there who think the answer to their health lies only in their MD's hands, which may result in missed healing opportunities, worsening medical conditions, or serious side effects that end up doing more harm than their initial diagnosis.

I must reiterate that I believe that medical doctors have some of the answers, but certainly not all of them. Each type of healer studies something specific, and not one person is an expert in all facets of healing. This is one of the reasons why it's so important to be open to seeing a variety of doctors. My advice to you is to keep an open mind to an array of solutions, get to know your own body, and listen to what it is telling you. Do as much of your own research as possible, then act on a combination of those collective insights to find the answer to recovery.

The time spent with my dad allowed us to discuss our different points of view around health care, and I'm happy that he is becoming more open to the idea of seeking treatment outside of an MD's office. However, what I treasured the most about my dad's solo visit was that it allowed me to bond more closely with him.

Loving Conversations

For the most part, the people around you (including your doctors) want what's best for you. They might express their concerns or opinions, but you are the one living with your condition. You must make informed decisions regarding your healing. This is your life — the only one you have — and you need to rise up and take accountability and responsibility for your healing. Just try to explain your rationale to those around you in a loving but firm way.

CHAPTER 9

LEARN TO SPEAK UP

"Change starts with showing up and letting ourselves be seen."
~Brené Brown

I have found that learning to trust your gut and speak up for yourself is an instrumental part of the self-healing process. It's not enough to just know what you can implement in your life without having a voice to express this to your loved ones, medical practitioners, and other support systems.

I consider myself extremely fortunate to have grown up in such a loving, close-knit family with siblings and parents who truly support one another. I was always encouraged in my efforts and made to feel special. Despite this loving and supportive system, I was never one to voice my thoughts unless I felt very comfortable with those around me. In addition to my inherently shy nature, I attended a Catholic grade school. While I actually loved my experiences at this school, for the most part, I learned that there was a definite way to behave if you eventually wanted to end up in Heaven. So I worked hard to say the right things and behave properly.

I remember starting some days at school sitting at my desk with my hands folded in prayer, saying to myself that it was a new day and that I would be "good" starting now. Unfortunately, my good behavior never seemed to last more than 24 hours, according to holy standards. It was very important to respect and listen to my teachers. They had the final word and weren't questioned, even if their views or behaviors didn't always seem to make sense or align with what they taught.

As I grew into adulthood, I continued to respect and listen to authority figures, including dentists, doctors, and teachers. I automatically assumed that they knew what was best for me. After my college years, I found myself working in a restaurant as a waitress and almost lost that job because I was so reserved. Luckily, management held off on their decision and gave me enough time to show that I could be vocal. It was actually this job that helped me begin to overcome my shyness. I was forced to wait on and speak to many different customers each day. As a result, I learned that every person shares basic commonalities, no matter their status in life. I flexed this social muscle during every shift as I was exposed to a variety of people, gradually becoming less intimidated with each conversation and encounter. This job represented a small turning point for me.

When I became a single parent in my twenties, I started to strengthen my voice even further. I knew I was going to keep this baby and raise him on my own, and I made that abundantly clear to those around me. I soon realized that it was noticeably easier to speak up when I was doing it on behalf of another human being, rather than for myself.

When my son was about two years old, I met the man I would marry – a man who would later adopt my son as his own. Relationships are complicated, so I'll just say that over the years I began losing myself in a marriage that clearly wasn't serving either of us. After coming to terms with the reality of our relationship, I finally made one of the toughest decisions I've ever had to make – divorcing my husband.

This became the second turning point for me. Once I made that major decision for myself and saw that I would be able to survive all the ramifications that followed, it empowered me to build on the newfound freedom that came from trusting my own judgement in order to thrive. Although that time in my life took a great emotional toll on me and my family, it also promoted great inner strength, resilience, and personal and spiritual growth.

I believe that my marriage taught me many lessons. Among those lessons was learning to be vocal and express my thoughts and opinions — something that would serve me well further into the future when I would need to become my own greatest advocate for my health.

Exercise: Raising Your Voice

If you struggle to speak up in any aspect of your life, it can be helpful to keep some predetermined phrases in your pocket. These could be something as simple as, "From my perspective, what you're saying is…". While it may seem simple, this type of preparation can open the floodgates for positive dialogue and act as a buffer between what you've heard and how you feel about it. When doing this, keep a few ground rules in mind:

1. Speaking up for yourself doesn't mean losing compassion for the person to whom you're speaking.
2. "No" is a complete answer, and you don't need to overexplain yourself. Sometimes, this only gives others ammunition to convince you out of your feelings or thoughts.
3. Be clear about what you think and feel. Don't muddle your words, but speak slowly and consciously.

CHAPTER 10

Become a Super Sleuth

"Those who have no time for healthy eating will sooner or later have to find the time for illness."

~Edward Stanley

Now we need to look at the health links between what you might be battling and the potential underlying causes. When you're able to rule certain things out — or in — it can serve as a good foundation on which you can begin building your healing journey. Let's start off with anemia and iron.

Anemia & Iron

"When people are working to manage an autoimmune or chronic condition, they typically focus on an anti-inflammatory diet and protocol. However, one often overlooked dealbreaker to getting better is anemia. Anemia is a deal breaker to recovery because it means your cells are not getting enough oxygen. Without oxygen, recovery and repair can't happen." (4)

It's important to get your iron levels tested. While it's beneficial to have an anti-inflammatory diet in place, you also want to make sure you're not diminishing your level of iron intake as a result. One of the most common misconceptions is that you can only get healthy doses of iron from meat. While meat can be an excellent source of protein, it certainly isn't the only good source of iron. You can find iron in a lot of wonderful leafy greens. The huge benefit of getting your iron from greens as opposed to meat lies in the type of iron that you're getting. The heme iron found in meat is readily absorbed by the body. While most people would assume this is a good thing, it actually isn't. If you're taking in too much heme iron, your body doesn't know when enough is enough. It will continue absorbing that iron even if you're way past the threshold for iron intake, which can eventually lead to health complications like heart disease. On the other hand, the non-heme iron found in plants is filtered out of your body once you've reached your capacity for iron intake. Simply put, you can eat as many leafy greens as you like without there ever being a detrimental effect.

According to Dr. Michael Greger, "It is commonly thought that those who eat plant-based diets may be more prone to iron deficiency, but it turns out that they're no more likely to suffer from iron deficiency anemia than anybody else. This may be because not only do those eating meat-free diets tend to get more fiber, magnesium, and vitamins like A, C, and E, but they also get more iron." (5)

So, load up on kale, spinach, and other leafy greens to supplement your iron levels, and keep away from foods and beverages that can deplete iron, such as dairy foods and foods rich in tannins (like coffee, tea, and chocolate).

Here are some healthy substitutes for the following:
- Cow's milk: Have the purest coconut or almond milk you can find without carrageenan or guar gums. (I prefer Native Forest Organic Unsweetened Simple Coconut Milk.)
- Chocolate: Limit yourself to an occasional dark chocolate with a high cacao concentration. (I like unsweetened Santa Barbara chocolates melted over fruit.)

- Black tea and coffee: Opt for herbal teas and nutrient-dense smoothies, or work on your sleep cycle to feel more refreshed without the caffeine boost.

Next, you'll need to address the issue of low cortisol, if that's a problem for your personally.

The Consequences of Low Cortisol

If you struggle with low cortisol, you may experience:
- Weakness
- Fatigue
- Low blood pressure
- Vomiting
- Dizzy spells
- Loss of consciousness (in severe cases)

If you experience any of these symptoms, it's important to get your cortisol levels tested. Once your doctor has confirmed that your cortisol is low, the next step is to figure out what's affecting your adrenal glands' cortisol production. The treatment your doctor recommends will be, in large part, determined by the source of the problem. Let's have a look at some sources of low cortisol:
- Adrenal fatigue: This occurs when your body can't cope with daily stress, poor diet, lack of sleep, or emotional trauma. As a result, your adrenal glands become overloaded and ineffective.
- Primary adrenal insufficiency (Addison's disease): This condition develops when your adrenal glands are damaged and therefore can't function properly to produce cortisol. It can be caused by an autoimmune disease, tuberculosis, an underlying infection of the adrenal glands, certain cancers in the adrenal glands, or bleeding into the adrenal glands.

- Secondary adrenal insufficiency: This occurs when the pituitary gland, which produces a hormone that stimulates the adrenal glands, is diseased. The adrenal glands themselves may be healthy, but they won't be able to produce enough cortisol if they aren't being properly stimulated by the pituitary gland. If you've been prescribed corticosteroids and stop taking them suddenly, secondary adrenal insufficiency can occur.

Every hormone that we have in our bodies is there for a reason. While it's not good to have high cortisol levels, it's no better to have low levels of this hormone. To ensure you have balanced cortisol levels, try the following tips:

- Practice mindfulness meditation and deep-breathing techniques.
- Move your body and stretch as much as you can throughout the day. If your job requires you to sit in front of a computer all day, be sure to take lots of walk breaks.
- Get as much natural sunlight as possible.
- Maintain consistent waking and sleeping times (even on weekends).
- Avoid backlit devices like laptops, computer screens, TVs, and phones for at least three hours before bed.
- Eat balanced meals that are primarily rooted in whole foods.

CHAPTER 11

MORE MUCH-NEEDED FAMILY SUPPORT

"Remember, you have been criticizing yourself for years and it hasn't worked. Try approving of yourself and see what happens."
~Louise L. Hay

My mom arrived within a few hours of my dad's departure. Having her at the house provided me with the emotional support that I really needed at that moment. She has always been so supportive of me and whatever goal I am trying to achieve, and I definitely feel the unconditional love she has for me. We can talk about anything and everything or watch our favorite shows together and, somehow, everything feels like it's going to be alright.

The following week, my brother arrived, eager to help in any way he could. Despite his own health issues related to Crohn's disease, he powered through a variety of projects around the house, including repairing a faulty refrigerator that had had been leaking on my wood floor. I expressed how amazing it was that he was able to successfully tackle so many tasks and do them well, sharing how appreciative I was for his help. Despite the quality of his work and the amount he achieved during his visit, he seemed temporarily stuck on the fact that it took him a couple tries to repair the refrigerator. He was listening to the critical voice inside his own head and becoming frustrated with himself in the process — something that I've realized we all do to varying degrees. We all need to be kinder to ourselves and appreciate the positive things that we bring to our world. As I once read, we should speak to ourselves as if we were small children. How would you respond to the seven-year-old you?

Exercise: Loving Your Inner Child

I would like you to take a moment to pen a letter to your seven-year-old self. What would you say to them if they were battling this health condition? How would you reassure them?

Going forward, do your best to speak to your adult self with the same patience, compassion, and understanding whenever the inner critic inside of you arises and attempts to thwart your valiant efforts to elevate your life. While this can be particularly helpful in your healing journey, it can also extend to every facet of your life.

*

If there's one thing that you should take away from all of this, it's the understanding that true healing begins when you're able to commit to a more loving vibration. From there, it will be far easier to determine what needs to be eliminated from your spiritual and physical environment.

In fact, after my brother had left, I decided to do a physical detox with a colon cleanse, followed by a liver cleanse, purchased online through the Global Healing Center. The website mentions that you should do the colon cleanse first to ensure that the proper pathway is open before you start eliminating toxins through your liver and kidneys. After completing these cleanses, I felt good — physically and emotionally.

CHAPTER 12

A Heavy Metal Cleanse

"In a new field called epigenetics, we are discovering how meditation, joy, compassion, forgiveness, and the food we eat can switch on the genes that create health and switch off the genes that create disease."
~Alberto Villoldo

I decided to start addressing the overload of heavy metals in my body, which had shown up in previous urine testing with my naturopath, by starting a 30-day heavy metal detox protocol through the Global Healing Center. In conjunction with that, I also consumed specific ingredients at the recommendation of the Medical Medium. Each item, listed below, supposedly has its own unique ability to help clear toxins. By working in harmony with one another, they have the power to pull toxins from your brain and bones in order to fully eliminate them from your body. Now let's walk through those ingredients.

Daily Heavy Metal Cleanse Ingredients
1. 2 tsp. of spirulina (spirulina from Hawaii is preferable)
2. 1-2 tsp. of barley grass powder
3. ½ cup to 1 cup of cilantro
4. At least 1 cup of wild Maine blueberries (they need to be wild!)
5. 2 tbsp. of Atlantic Dulse flakes

Whether you combine these ingredients into one daily drink or take them separately throughout the day, it's important that you take them all within a 24-hour period to benefit from their collective ability to eliminate heavy metals from your body (according to the Medical Medium). Since the supplement industry is unregulated, it is important to find clean supplements without harmful additives or unnecessary fillers. I suggest considering reputable brands such as Thorne or BioPure and buying directly from the source (not a third party).

During the month of April, I scheduled a few chiropractic treatments to keep my body aligned. After all this time on crutches, my body had started to make adjustments that weren't necessarily in its best interest. I also had a physical therapy appointment, at which the practitioner said she saw improvements from the last time that I was in her office. She noticed that I wasn't quite as protective of my foot anymore and that I wasn't constantly rubbing it as I had done in the past — a habit I had picked up to warm it due to the lack of circulation that the inflammation had caused. I was also able to walk lightly on my right foot without the aid of crutches. She was happy to see this because she had initially been worried about how my inactivity would affect my right leg. The muscle mass in my right leg had been atrophying, and neither of us wanted that to continue.

NOTE: Muscular atrophy is the wasting away of muscular tissue. This can occur if there is little to no circulation to the area or if muscles lose their nerve supply.

I decided to celebrate my April birthday that year with what I called a "friendship lunch." Rather than celebrating **myself**, I wanted to celebrate my friends for all the wonderful support they had provided over the last several months. Each friend was given a personal cupcake, complete with a candle so they could make their own wish, along with a card expressing what I appreciated most about them. I also gave them each a mug with a gift card in it. Hopefully they all felt the love and gratitude I held for each of them!

Reiki: A First Encounter

Energy healing fascinates me, so I treated myself to a Reiki session and a shiatsu massage by a bodyworker named Yael. Following the treatment, Yael said that she could tell I had a lot of creative energy but that I needed to open the throat chakra and express myself. This statement rang especially true for me since I had been feeling a growing urge to express myself through photography but was having trouble with my overall confidence as well as speaking up about my pricing and packages. Whether the practitioner truly saw my energy or not, I can't say for sure, but her statement did give me something to contemplate. It can be difficult to get a definitive result from any type of energy healing, but I can say that I did feel quite peaceful during the process and that my foot stopped bothering me during the session. Some might say that the information she provided was somewhat generic, but it was exactly what I needed to hear at that moment in order to move forward. Your soul knows what you need, so remain open to all possibilities and you will hear the most pertinent information for **you**.

Determining Your Blockages

1. Your root chakra, which is at the base of your spine, may be blocked if you feel constantly fearful or worried. You might find yourself living with an inability to take action in your life. Meditating and walking barefoot on the grass are great ways to release or open your root chakra.
2. Your sacral chakra, found in your lower back, may be blocked if you find yourself dealing with constant stress or emotional outbursts.

You might also find yourself overindulging in certain guilty pleasures in an attempt to regulate your mood. Swimming and aromatherapy work well when it comes to unblocking your sacral chakra.

3. The solar plexus chakra, located near your belly button, is your source of power. When this chakra is blocked, you might struggle with crippling self-doubt. Getting a good amount of daily sun and practicing yoga and meditation are great remedies for a blocked solar plexus chakra.
4. The heart chakra is exactly where it says it is. When your heart chakra is blocked, you might find that you are less compassionate and unable to forgive. You might also experience heart problems. Eat lots of leafy greens and spend as much time as possible with the people you love to unblock this chakra.
5. The throat chakra supports your ability to communicate and express your creativity. You might find that you experience frequent issues that arise from miscommunication if your throat chakra is blocked. There are also physical symptoms of this blockage, such as a stiff neck and sore throat. Eat lots of healthy, organic, blue foods and meditate frequently.
6. The third eye chakra, located between your brows, controls your perception. You may experience a disconnect from your sense of intuition, as well as brain fog and dizzy spells, if this chakra is blocked. Essential oils, such as frankincense, are great for unblocking the third eye chakra. Massage some into your hands to uplift yourself throughout the day.
7. Finally, there is the crown chakra, which sits atop your head. When you are too attached to material things, your crown chakra can become blocked. This can make you feel apathetic, as if you've lost your passion and drive for life. Spend as much time in nature as

possible and burn scents like juniper around your home to get your balance back.

Rheumatologist Follow-Up

After my Reiki appointment, I had another appointment scheduled for the end of April with Dr. S. I let him know that I didn't want to go on Humira, the biologic drug that was suggested by the other rheumatologist, and instead wanted to get off all medication completely. He agreed that I could forgo the Humira but advised me to stay on the methotrexate for the time being while continuing to decrease my prednisone dosage gradually.

Reflecting on the content I read in *The Road Back*, I began to wonder if I could heal my autoimmune issues by living in the warm climate of Arizona, as the authors mentioned. Since I had family in Tucson, it wasn't a difficult decision to live there for the month of May, just to determine if it would be beneficial to my health. Even though I would be coming from California — a place that already had a consistent barometric pressure and warm temperature — and my condition had been reclassified from rheumatoid arthritis to ankylosing spondylitis, it was still worth a shot. My dad flew out to accompany my dog, Lucy, and me on our road trip to our temporary home in Tucson.

A New Home for Healing

In May of 2016, I was still reliant on the crutches and knee scooter. I could just about get a sock over my foot, but not a shoe. I tried to remain grateful during this time. The thing is, you can't be upset and grateful at the same time, so each day I try to think of things to appreciate. I created a gratitude list based on the simple joys that I experienced during my first couple of days in Tucson. You can use this as inspiration for your own list.

My Gratitude List:
- Shopped at Crate & Barrel with my parents and stopped to get a healthy juice drink on the way home. So grateful to spend this time with my mom and dad…and for the healthy drink.
- Meditated this morning, which is always peaceful and calming.
- Finalized plans for my friend to visit from the East Coast.
- Appreciated having Lucy, my Shih Tzu, snuggled up next to me.
- Soaked in an Epsom salt and lavender bath. It helped me relax, sleep better, and sooth the swelling in my foot.
- Found a gluten-free, dairy-free chocolate with cacao, which served as a guilt-free way to satisfy my sweet tooth.

I had settled into my temporary rental space in Tucson quite nicely and had been able to walk around the condo a little bit without crutches. I began to realize just how much progress I had made since the beginning of my healing journey. By May, I was able to walk around the condo on my right heel more quickly without the use of crutches, although I still had to avoid putting pressure on the ball of my inflamed foot.

Navigating Negativity

While trying to maintain an attitude of gratitude, it's more than likely that you'll hear something, see something, or experience something that throws you off course. While I was in Tucson, I heard some unsettling news, and I found myself feeling weighed down by it. It brought a sharp jab of negativity into my life at a time when I was trying to maintain a deep sense of gratitude. Over the span of the previous five months, I had made a big point of eliminating any negativity around me. I wouldn't allow doctors to say anything pessimistic about my condition and I didn't watch any news on TV. I found that, for the most part, insulating myself from the outside world was the only way that I could completely avoid negativity from others. Although my conscious efforts to shut out the outside noise did brighten my mood, my mindset, and my overall outlook on life, I found that this approach wasn't sustainable for the long term.

The tiniest and seemingly most inconsequential thoughts can affect your whole being, for better or worse, which is why it's so important to be careful of what we put in our minds and bodies, as well as what we allow to stay.

Following this tiny blip in my time of endless optimism, I started to feel contemplative, bored, and separated from the rest of the world. I felt alone and unsure of my higher purpose, and I was desperate to get back to the loving feeling that I had experienced so deeply in the first couple months of the year. I knew that I needed to be doing something creative and connecting with other people to relieve my boredom and feel happy and fulfilled. After a few days of dwelling on my path forward, I decided to write down some pursuits that would make me happy, eventually coming up with an expansive list of ideas. Although I was experiencing what felt like depression, I think this mental weight was actually what I refer to as "soul repression." I wasn't tapped into my purpose.

I decided to explore the Hay House Summit online. I love most of the authors that Hay House publishes, and this virtual summit offered a number of speakers each day that you could listen to for free for a limited time. I randomly chose to listen to the Soul Coach, Rha Goddess, who spoke about something called "the shaking before the awakening." She hit on just what I needed to hear that day. I had been trying to pave my career path and pinpoint my passion, and she offered a guided process for determining your purpose and contribution to the world.

During the summit, I also listened to a talk by Dr. Alberto Villoldo, a medical anthropologist, psychologist, and shaman who studied the spiritual practices of the people of the Andes and the Amazon for more than 30 years. During his time at San Francisco State University, he also founded the Biological Self-Regulation Laboratory, which was dedicated to studying how the mind creates psychosomatic health issues and diseases.

I loved his lecture so much that I went out and bought his book, *One Spirit Medicine: Ancient Ways to Ultimate Wellness*, the next day. Shortly after that, I checked out his website and decided to make a deposit for a week-long healing retreat hosted by him in Chile. It was set to take place in December, and I was thrilled to be going on a trip that represented the perfect adventure for me. The retreat offered the opportunity to experience many different healing modalities, including shaman energy medicine sessions, glutathione treatments, oxygen therapy, and much more. The best part was that we would be taking part in all of this while indulging in healthy, carefully prepared meals and basking in the endless beauty of Chile. Normally, I might wish for time to pass more quickly in anticipation of an exciting adventure ahead, but I truly enjoyed each day leading up to the trip with a renewed sense of gratitude.

Another synchronicity popped into my view on the same day that I had booked the week-long retreat. I had been so caught up with trying to figure out my purpose, and I just so happened to come across a short clip featuring Steven Spielberg. He spoke about "listening to the whisper in your ear" when figuring out your career path. This is yet another example of how putting your questions, desires, or intentions out into the world can bring you the answers you need most. When you ask the

Universe for something, be sure your eyes and ears are open to receive the answers!

Laughter Is the Best Medicine

My oldest brother stopped by before my visit in Tucson came to an end, and we had the chance to hang out for a bit before heading out to dinner with our parents. There are many people in my life, and each relationship seems to provide something different. In my brother's case, I find that he's someone who will always joke with me and appreciate my humor. Even if something in my life goes badly, I can retell the story in a funny way, and he'll give me the perfect response — a laugh — rather than pitying me.

CHAPTER 13

Reading Breakthroughs

"Set yourself free from the past. Set yourself free from the expectations of others. Set yourself free to simply be yourself, and you will soar higher than you've ever dreamed."

~Cary G. Weldy

Although I didn't notice any improvements in my condition while I was in Arizona and continued to rely on the knee scooter everywhere I went, I was grateful that I had at least gotten to spend some more quality time with my family, whose presence alone provided a different kind of healing.

On the way back home to San Jose, I read a magazine article that detailed the process of smudging your home with sage. Smudging, a method of removing stagnant or heavy energy, has also been proven to cleanse the air in your environment. If you'd like to try it out for yourself, follow the steps below.

Smudging with Sage

You will need:
- White sage
- An abalone shell
- A feather
- Matches

To get started, you'll need to light your smudging stick over an abalone shell and then fan it away from yourself with a feather as you walk around your home. Be sure to walk into each room and smudge the area thoroughly by moving from corner to corner. You can state your affirmations aloud or in your mind to put out positive intentions as you make your way around each room. Allow the sage to clear out as much negative energy as possible, making sure to keep the windows open and fully extinguish the embers from the sage before storing it away once you're done.

When I think of how I found this smudging method in a magazine, it reminds me of how much I love to read. So many of my childhood memories revolve around reading. When I was little, I spent hours reading the *Nancy Drew* books and many others, always seeming to find a sense of peace within the walls of libraries and bookstores. So, throughout my healing journey, I turned to my favorite pastime and devoured books that were spiritual in nature, related to healing, or centered around personal transformation. I searched unwaveringly for inspiration to heal more completely.

While reading *The Untethered Soul: The Journey Beyond Yourself* by Michael A. Singer, a particular quote stood out to me: "When you truly awaken spiritually, you realize you are caged. You wake up and realize that you can hardly move in there. You're constantly hitting the limits of your comfort zone. You see that you're afraid to tell people what you really think. You see that you're too self-conscious to freely express yourself." (6)

I began to think more about ways that I might fully express myself at all times in the future. I tend to censor myself in many ways, whether it's holding back my sense of humor until I know someone better or hiding a big part of myself by not sharing my views on health or spiritual beliefs. I was even mindful of what I said to specific friends, knowing that certain beliefs weren't "their thing." I was cautious about coming off as odd or crazy, believing that censoring myself was the simplest way to ward off any potential rejection. It's the times when I'm around those people with whom I can't fully be myself that I feel unhappy, dissatisfied, or depressed.

On the contrary, it's the times that I've listened to my heart and intuition, no matter how unconventional my choices may have seemed, that I have gained the most reward — emotionally, physically, spiritually, and even financially. When I live life on my terms and feel free to express myself completely, I feel liberated. When I ignore all the fear-based advice of others, I'm able to live a life that fulfills me and gives me purpose. This all allows me to contribute to the evolution of this planet in my own unique way.

Have you ever put a puzzle together, only to discover at the very end that you're missing a piece or two? If so, you can probably understand the frustration of not being able to see the "full picture." Similarly, if we're not able to share our own unique qualities, talents, and insights while on this earth, we may be withholding key pieces to life's collective puzzle, potentially preventing others from benefiting from our gifts and furthering their own growth.

I'll leave you with another quote from *The Untethered Soul*: "Going beyond means going beyond the borders of the cage. There should be no cage. The soul is infinite. It is free to expand everywhere. It is free to experience all of life. This can only happen when you are willing to face reality without mental boundaries." (7)

Now, before we move on to the next chapter, let's look at how you can free your soul.

Exercise: Freeing Your Soul

1. In keeping with what I spoke of in the previous chapter, I want you to place incredible importance on how much laughter you engage in daily. Find a funny comic strip or comedy film, or just search for corny jokes on the internet. When you laugh from the pits of your stomach, you can set your soul free.
2. Cultivate an inner circle of people who appreciate the genuine and uncensored version of yourself. Living your most authentic self will relax your body and uncage your soul.
3. If you haven't started this yet, begin journaling everything that you're grateful for daily, no matter how small. Life can be lived in full color when you don't take the little things for granted.

CHAPTER 14

RELEASING WHAT NO LONGER SERVES YOU

After coming back home from Arizona, I was able to walk around more frequently without crutches. Although I still couldn't apply full pressure to the ball of my right foot, the inflammation had gone down and I had gradually reduced my prednisone intake from 40 mg to 7.5 mg per day.

Not all the news was positive, however, as I had been losing large handfuls of hair every time I showered. My hairdresser was the second person to notice how dramatically my hair had thinned over the previous two months. The methotrexate seemed to be taking its toll.

Wanderlust had now kicked in at full force, and I decided to book a trip to Bali in November with a spiritual educator and author. I was drawn to the spiritual healing journey that she promised, and I was excited by the prospect of participating in all of the activities being offered, which included visits to the elephant sanctuary, a session with a well-known healer, lodging at Ketut's place — yes, THAT Ketut from Elizabeth Gilbert's *Eat, Pray, Love* novel — healthy food choices, and the chance to connect with a group of people who were also on a spiritual healing venture.

Time to Declutter

By June 10, I was able to exchange the sock on my foot for a flip-flop — a small victory! By this time, I was making a daily effort to keep my house clear of clutter, not just for the sake of mobility but for the spiritual, physical, and psychological benefits of living in a decluttered space.

I find that the decluttering process raises my energy levels and gives me more clarity and motivation. If I'm ever feeling "stuck," the first thing I do is clear clutter and get organized. I find that it allows new energy to come into the cleared space. When you hold on to a lot of old possessions, you're also holding on to those past experiences and the energy that accompanies them. The only way to move forward and create something new is to clear out the clutter of your past, mentally and physically. Only keep the material things that you **love** or really need, relinquishing any items associated with guilt or unpleasant memories that you hope to leave in the past.

I have found that the best way to declutter is to pull everything out of a closet or space and then physically hold each item close to you. This allows you to gauge if the item is something you immediately resonate with or love. If you know immediately you don't want it, put it in the "donate" pile. If you aren't sure, quickly put it in a separate "maybe" pile. Once you finish the process, put all of the items that are a definite "yes" back into the closet or space and take a moment to notice how it feels energetically.

You'll usually discover that you're able to let go of the "maybe" pile more easily at that point. You don't need the energy of guilt or regret or a "coulda, woulda, shoulda" mindset weighing you down. You'll be amazed at how great you feel walking into your home and basking in the positive energy that comes from surrounding yourself with only those things that make you happy! I typically finish off this process by burning some sage throughout my house, which cleanses the air and frees my space of any stagnant or heavy energy.

If you're looking to free yourself from your own physical and mental clutter, a favorite book of mine that I recommend is Karen Kingston's *Clear Your Clutter with Feng Shui.*

Exercise: Your Declutter Diary

1. Make a list of all of the items, bad memories, or even negative people you may want to release from your life.
2. Think about whether anything in your home reminds you of negative periods in your life.
3. Now, begin your decluttering process, as highlighted above.
4. If there are items that have a negative effect on you (perhaps remind you of a painful past), start making plans to replace them. Start a little fund to prepare for any replacements, then get rid of the old items, one by one.

CHAPTER 15

Physical & Spiritual Detoxing

"The meaning of life is to find your gift. The purpose of life is to give it away."

~Pablo Picasso

Mid-June brought with it the need to continue cleansing myself on a physical and spiritual level. You might find that you need to detox quite frequently when you move through your healing journey. This is because it's quite easy for even the most microscopic levels of negative energy or toxicity to creep in and stay as you move toward an elevated and healthier way of living.

I had been gathering the necessary supplements for the 30-day detox laid out in Alberto Villoldo's *One Spirit Medicine*. Detoxing and rejuvenating my body had become my two favorite activities! I followed Villoldo's entire protocol, which included an 18-hour fast from sugar and carbs as well as a variety of supplements.

I decided to schedule another session with Yael, the bodyworker, for a combination of shiatsu, Reiki, and theta therapies. During the session, my head felt quite heavy. Yael said she was feeling, energetically, the need for me to communicate my feelings with others, before letting any negative emotions build up. I made a mental note to be more forthcoming with my feelings going forward and signed up through Yael to become certified in Reiki I, with the intention of becoming a self-healer and enhancing my intuitive side.

As I continued my June regimen of cleansing my space, I had my rugs and chairs professionally cleaned along with the windows. I cleared out some clutter and, as usual, found it uplifting to get things organized, cleaned, and cleared out. I followed this up with a sage-burning session throughout my house while surrounding myself with Light and Love, asking the Spirit to remove any stagnant or negative energy from the space. I made a request that the rooms be filled with peace, love, joy, happiness, and a higher vibrational energy.

When Self-Love Dwindles

Around this time, I was finding it somewhat difficult to focus during my meditations. I also found myself censoring everything I said, over-analyzing my thoughts, and allowing a sense of uncertainty to seep back into my life. Over time, those feelings that I harbored caused me to question my career path, my passion, and my overall purpose in life.

I ruminated over my value as a parent and worried that people didn't know the authentic me. Feeling insecure is uncomfortable, but I was determined not to retreat into my own secluded world, despite how much more comfortable it may have seemed in comparison. I knew that this would just be a temporary way of avoiding any unwanted emotions. I preferred to feel surrounded and strengthened by the power of love, just as I had back in January. I had felt an overwhelming sense of connection and love at that time, which I was eager to share with everyone I met. Nothing could dampen my spirits during that six-week period, and I wanted to be blessed with that feeling once again.

I believe that what I needed most in those moments was a big dose of self-love. I needed to provide myself with a sense of value and determine my own self-worth without the input of other people. I've found that the best way to enhance self-love is by finding work that makes you happy and allows you to incorporate the creative and spiritual sides of yourself. That, as well as surrounding myself with those people with whom I can truly be myself, works wonders for me. Ever since becoming reliant on crutches and a knee scooter, I hadn't been able to function as a paid photographer. Now that I was able to put some pressure on my right foot, I felt a need to shoot a practice photo session with my friend, Hailey, to refresh my photography skills and test my ability to move around the studio. Our practice session went well, as I was able to tolerate the time spent on my feet. I realized that I enjoyed capturing the emotions and personalities of women in particular. I told Hailey that I wanted to re-center my business around photographing women — artsy, creative, sensual images — rather than continuing my previous pursuit of corporate headshot sessions. I found that I preferred the creative freedom, personal connections, and emotionally healing aspect of boudoir photography, discovering a newfound sense of fulfillment in encouraging women, myself included, to be confident in their own skin.

Exercise: Finding Your Purpose

Finding your purpose is no small feat. You need to be able to suspend your ego and look at your life with a growth mindset. Some people are convinced that time has passed them by and that they're too old to start a new career or change the trajectory of their lives. I'm here to tell you that nothing could be further from the truth. You are worthy at any age. You can reinvent yourself a thousand times over. You only get this one precious life. Live it! You can start to conjure your purpose by doing the following:
1. Develop a growth mindset so that you can allow yourself to experience new things.

2. Become part of a community (or a few)! You just might discover a new passion that you never knew existed.
3. Spend as much time as possible with people who inspire you.
4. Give back to those around you, expecting nothing in return.
5. Create a vision for your life. Consider it a personal mission statement.

Now, you might be wondering how to develop a growth mindset. Luckily, it's simple! All it requires is an inherent belief in yourself and the embodiment of the following perspective:

- Challenges help me to rise up and grow.
- I can master any new skill I set my mind to.
- I have a desire to learn.
- There is no such thing as failure. There are only lessons.
- I can draw inspiration from others.

If you can focus on cultivating this mindset, you can conquer anything that comes your way!

This way of thinking has truly helped me to feel more positive and, by the end of June, my appointment with the naturopath had produced equally positive results. My blood test results showed positive numbers, except for low ferritin, which I then chose to supplement. I was elated to see some promising changes and knew that all the efforts I was making to regain my health were starting to work.

I took a stool test, which would reveal if I had parasites and candida overgrowth. Parasites can trigger autoimmune conditions and often impede your recovery if they go unchecked, according to the 1991 article Parasitic infection and autoimmunity as published by the National Center for Biotechnology Information. (8)

It makes one wonder. If this has been known for so long, why isn't more being done about it?

CHAPTER 16

ENERGETIC SHIFTS

"The moment you change your perception, is the moment you rewrite the chemistry of your body."

~Dr. Bruce H. Lipton

By July 6, I had begun my Reiki I class. It was interesting to learn and practice this form of healing on the other students in the class. The instructor worked on my throat chakra while the other students worked on my sacral chakra, as I had requested. At one point during the session, I felt the instructor's hands move from my throat chakra to my heart chakra. I happily welcomed the unexpected transition since I was hoping to have that chakra worked on as well.

When I opened my eyes, I told the instructor that I had felt her shift to the heart chakra, but she surprisingly insisted that she had never moved her hands from their place at my throat chakra. I found this strange since I had vividly felt a sensation of heavy hands being placed over my heart. She explained that the energy knows where it needs to go and moves there on its own.

I then practiced Reiki on a willing subject, under the supervision of the instructor. The subject had his eyes closed as I held my hands several inches above his throat chakra and implemented the Reiki practices. Suddenly, the man called out that he felt tightness around his throat and asked me to lighten my grip, even though my hands were not physically on his throat at all. This was just further proof to me that this type of energy healing was powerful.

NOTE: Some hospitals in the United States currently offer patients Reiki as an optional part of their treatment plan to accelerate healing and reduce anxiety both pre – and post operatively.

After finishing my instruction, I began performing Reiki sessions on myself. I purchased a book by Gail Thackray that offers clear-cut directions for performing Reiki on others or yourself. This was a perfect supplement to the class instruction that I had received.

I went to my physical therapy appointment, and the therapist was noticeably surprised by my improvement and my ability to get around much more freely. By this point, I was still taking methotrexate but had successfully decreased my prednisone dosage to 2.5 mg.

Having medical practitioners walk your journey to self-healing with you might just help the next person they treat. When they're able to see convincing evidence of your progress, this can spur a movement that helps countless others.

CHAPTER 17

PROGRESS & SETBACKS

As July progressed, I began to see more positive changes in my life. I received my Reiki II certificate, which meant I was now officially able to practice on others and myself. I walked into my local hair salon with only a slight limp, no longer confined by the crutches that had carried me into my previous appointment. I was still losing my hair due to the effects of the methotrexate but had now gotten myself completely off prednisone!

By the beginning of August, I had received my test results back from the naturopath. The heavy metal results showed that many metals, including mercury, had decreased in my system. However, the lead had doubled, and a handful of other metals, including arsenic, barium, and nickel, had also increased. I wasn't sure if they were elevated because I had detoxed metals during the month of May, allowing them to be drawn out of my bones and brain but not fully released from my bloodstream. Maybe I was continuing to be exposed to an unidentified source of lead. I knew it wasn't coming from tap water or from the paint in my home since I drank bottled water and had replaced my old doors and repainted my house with non-toxic paint during a remodel several years prior.

The stool test results revealed that I didn't have parasites or candida. They also showed very low inflammation, indicating that I didn't have a "leaky gut". I wasn't certain if the low dose of prednisone that I was on at the time of the test had affected the inflammation marker or not.

Other results showed signs of toxic overload in my body, and I suspected that methotrexate was the culprit. The verdict: more digestive enzymes and better probiotics!

Ways to Raise Your Energetic Vibration

I woke up with a heavy heart on most mornings, feeling anxious and spiritually disconnected. However, I found several methods that raised my spirits and reinvigorated my excitement for life's many possibilities. I incorporated the habits below in my daily routine to raise my vibrational frequency at this time.

- Meditation
- A good exercise routine
- Talking to a friend or close family member
- Thinking about upcoming events or travel opportunities
- Envisioning exciting future plans, even if they seemed far-fetched

In order to bolster my efforts to eliminate the lead and any other toxins that had accumulated in my body, I began a detox protocol through my naturopath. This particular protocol consisted of taking liver support supplements along with HM Chelate, a carefully crafted formula that supports immune defenses while bolstering your body's natural ability to release toxins.

I had difficulty sleeping at night, but I found it beneficial to lay on an acupressure mat that I had placed on my bed. I also listened to meditation music while I practiced Reiki on myself. I tend to fall asleep quickly this way.

CHAPTER 18

Adventures & Medical Diaries

"Once you make a decision, the Universe conspires to make it happen."

~Ralph Waldo Emerson

One of my favorite places to visit is the quaint and quiet town of Carmel, California. When I want to celebrate a special occasion or just spend some time with my children, this is where I choose to go. With my son heading to Thailand for a couple of months and my daughter heading back to college, it felt like the perfect time to snap some last-minute family photos in this special place.

We came across a beautiful cypress tree and found a man nearby to take our photo. I struck up a conversation with him, and he shared that he visits this specific tree to honor his fiancé, who had passed away from breast cancer the previous year. They had both enjoyed coming with their dog to this very spot, so he continued the tradition by bringing her flowers and a soy latte to leave under the tree for her.

I shared that I believed she was there with him during these visits, and he said that he had felt her presence many times. I told him that I was sorry he wasn't able to spend more time with her and offered him the hug that she wasn't physically able to give. I later wondered if she had propelled me to have that conversation and offer that hug.

The weather in Carmel was perfect that day. Walking on the dunes was a little uncomfortable, but I managed to keep the weight off the sensitive part of my foot by walking backward up the hill. Sometimes you have to risk looking foolish for the sake of comfort!

When we returned home later that same day, I tuned in for Super Soul Sunday — an inspiring series hosted by Oprah Winfrey. The guest she interviewed that day was Gretchen Rubin, the author of *The Happiness Project*. Gretchen pointed out that most people want to be happy as a life goal but haven't spent the necessary time figuring out what exactly that means to them. Once you focus on it and clarify it, you can work toward it. This seems to be excellent advice for achieving any goal in life:

- Clarify it.
- Visualize it.
- And, I would also add…feel it.

More Signs

After reading Pam Grout's *E-Squared: Nine Do-It-Yourself Energy Experiments That Prove Your Thoughts Create Your Reality*, I decided to do my own little experiment and put a message out to the Universe, asking for a clear sign about the direction I should go in my career. I wanted to know whether I should stick with photography or explore another avenue. I said that I needed a sign by August 26, not feeling attached to any particular outcome when I made the request. I woke up the next morning to two emails requesting my photography services — one headshot and one boudoir. I hadn't received inquiries in months, especially since I had been off my feet for the past eight. I took it as a welcomed sign to continue with my photography business.

After this, it was time for another trip.

Ill-Health Abound

I was Missouri-bound to visit my aunt, with whom I share a close relationship. I cherish our time together because she is unwaveringly light-hearted, loves to laugh, and is always up for discussing anything and everything. One night, we stopped by my cousin's house for a wonderful dinner, finding serenity in their idyllic farmhouse home and the stunning stretches of land that surround it. As a striking sunset settled over their barn, the calming sound of crickets and conversation instantly filled me with peace.

My cousin's turbulent health was a stark contrast to the peace I felt there. She had been afflicted with many different conditions, including fibromyalgia and Sjogren's disease. It seems that everywhere I go, I find people who are suffering greatly from various autoimmune conditions and misdiagnosed symptoms. Therefore, it's not enough just to heal myself. I feel a great responsibility to help others avoid unnecessary pain and live a more empowered life.

On my return home to San Jose, I listened to a couple CDs by Mike Dooley, a metaphysical teacher and New York Times best-selling author. He spoke about how events come about in a sequence of unexpected ways and shared his belief that it benefits you to ask for the bigger picture without getting caught up in specific details. If you limit the Universe's gifts by putting restrictions on how they should be delivered to you, you may be closing yourself off from receiving something even greater. Dooley also spoke of taking action and being open to what is put in your path, which may take you on an unexpected detour to the ultimate outcome you desire.

Remember to take advantage of new opportunities as they present themselves, even if they seem unrelated to a specific goal you're focusing on.

This philosophy truly resonates with me. I've found that when I put a question out into the Universe, and don't attach myself to the answer or the way it will come to me, I always receive fantastic guidance in one form or another. Give the Universe free reign to answer your requests in unique and clever ways. You might be amazed at how creative it can be when you don't put limitations on it.

The Detox Paradox

When I got back from Missouri, I began another 30-day heavy metal cleanse, consuming the five specific ingredients listed in the Medical Medium's heavy metal detox protocol, while adding a detox protocol from the Global Healing Center into the mix for good measure.

The process of detoxing can often come with unwelcomed side effects known as a Herxheimer ("Herx") or "die-off" reactions that stem from the rapid elimination of bacteria, fungus, heavy metals, or parasites. If you experience nausea, headaches, or abdominal pain, make sure you're not detoxing too quickly — adjusting your supplement dosage as needed — and that you have the proper binders in place to carry the toxins out of your body as they're being released. Some typical binding supplements might include things like chlorella, activated charcoal, and bentonite clay. It's also important to stay well-hydrated and ensure that you're replacing any necessary minerals in your body that the detoxing process may be removing along with the toxic metals.

Keep in mind that sometimes things seemingly get worse before they get better. Don't get discouraged — these temporary side effects are often simply a part of the healing process that can serve as signs that you're on the right track.

In October, I started taking Rheumate, the prescription form of folic acid, as suggested by Dr. S. According to him, it was supposed to be absorbed more easily and would cut down on the negative side effects of the methotrexate. I noticed a significant improvement with my hair loss soon after, so it seemed to be having its intended impact.

The key takeaway from this is that you should find medication that works well with your own body. While some people hardly experience any side effects with certain medications, others might. Always follow your gut and try to find a medication regimen that works in your best interests.

At this point, another side effect surfaced. My foot had been acting up again, which could have been attributed to the consistent detoxing or the lack of discipline with my diet that past week.

*

If you can, try to keep a diary of your symptoms and flare-ups, as well as what you were taking during that time. It might provide insight into what works for your body and what doesn't. Also record environmental factors, such as changes in climate or location.

CHAPTER 19

A Visit to Ketut Liyer's Home

After weeks of anticipation, I was finally Bali-bound! The time had arrived to jet off to my healing retreat. I love traveling, especially when the destination revolves around healing, helping others, or honing my photography skills. My intention for going to Bali was to find healing for my body, as well as gain new insights to help me navigate my life more effectively.

Despite the rocky start of a missed flight and a two-hour delay for my ride upon arrival, I felt confident that my trip was headed in a positive direction. My Balinese driver was very friendly and, despite what seemed to be an accepted lack of any traffic rules, no one yelled or honked their horns in irritation. The Balinese people, in general, all seemed to exude such warmth and kindness. I learned that they typically begin their day at their home temples, worshipping and giving thanks. My personal opinion is that it would greatly benefit people in the United States if gratitude and meditation became a part of our daily routines from a young age.

Sadly, Ketut Liyer passed away several months before our visit, but his son was a very gracious host. On the night we arrived at Ketut's home, his son conducted a special ceremony to bring us luck and happiness, which he ended with an offer of a fruit platter and handmade bracelets. The following day, we visited a well-known Balinese healer, who we found on a platform in the center of a large courtyard surrounded by small temples. We each waited for our turn to see him, joining a line of people from across the world who were also eager to receive healing. When it was my turn to approach the healer, I sat down, and he placed his hands on both sides of my head. I felt what seemed like nails digging into one side of my scalp but later noticed that he didn't have long nails. He told me that I had anxiety, depression, and sadness, none of which I wanted to admit to but knew rang true. He then moved to my foot (the unafflicted one) and applied pressure to different places on my toes with something resembling a wooden chopstick. This seemed like a form of reflexology. He told me that I was missing passion and, when he wasn't sure if I was understanding, clarified with a simple, "It's been a long time." Embarrassing, but true! I laughed and jokingly asked if he could fix that. He wrapped up my session with some energy healing as I lay still and silent on the blanketed floor.

The following day, we visited a jungle temple that was known for its healing waters. I immediately plunged my right foot into them. It was in this place that our host gave us each an attunement similar to a Reiki energy healing. Once we got back to Ketut's home, I opted for one of their signature massage treatments, which was followed by a soothing soak in a rose petal bath. It was one of the best massages I've ever experienced, and I was able to sleep soundly that night.

The next day, we were educated about elephants and had the chance to see them up close as they bathed themselves in the pond. I was thrilled when we were told that we would later get to feed them their favorite fruit. This part of the trip was healing in its own unique way. Being connected to nature and to animals tends to relieve my stress and fill my heart with happiness.

We topped off our enchanting encounter with the elephants with a trip to a chocolate shop on the grounds, indulging in the various samples of savory chocolates they served.

In the late afternoon, we took advantage of something quite common in Bali. We made an appointment with a palm reader, who described my personality in detail. This was my reading:

1. **I do not like anyone leading me;**
2. **I have high creative energy and a strong mind and spirit;**
3. **My heart is weaker and that is why I am sensitive;**
4. **Moodiness is what holds me back;**
5. **I have so many different things I want to do, but I should zero in on only one of them for a year.**

He asked what those different endeavors might be, and I said:

1. Photography
2. Clearing clutter for people
3. Writing a book
4. Creating health and wellness retreats

He told me to devote my time to photography for at least one year before incorporating other pursuits. He noted that I had experienced three important romantic relationships, one of which was long. This was true, as I had only had two serious relationships before meeting the man I married. He said that I would have two more relationships coming in this lifetime. I would start a relationship, and the energy of that would last almost 10 years. He said this didn't necessarily mean that I would date this man for 10 years but simply that the energy of it would last that long. After those 10 years, that energy would clear away, opening the door for me to meet a man — my soul connection — who I would marry. He wouldn't give me any more details, claiming that I would get stuck trying to figure them out. In addition, he said that my mind was very open to new experiences and relationships but that I tend to take a while to get close to people.

His description of me was quite accurate, but I'll have to see if those two other relationships find their way to me.

Results Are In

My trip to Bali was truly a once-in-a-lifetime experience. It came at precisely the right moment, bringing a sense of restoration along with it. If you can, venture out and travel more, even if it's just around your state. Take in new sights and mingle with new people so you can broaden your perspective. After returning home from my transformative trip, I received my test results from the naturopath.

Toxic Metal Levels	Most of the heavy metals had decreased but the lead had actually doubled again. This may have been a result of all the detoxing I had been doing that year, since toxins can be pulled from the bones and organs but still show up in the blood before being fully expelled. Working with my naturopath, I continued to detox the lead.
Stool Test	The test revealed an uncommon gut infection, which you can acquire from certain types of foods that haven't been handled properly. The naturopath said my body would respond best to daily doses of uva ursi and berberis vulgaris.
Iron Levels	My iron levels were low once again. I began taking Ferrasorb iron capsules daily.
Neurotransmitters	My neurotransmitters, including adrenaline, GABA, noradrenaline, acetylcholine, dopamine, glutamine, serotonin, and endorphins, were low. This explained my lack of focus, fatigue, depression, and heightened perception of pain.

Micronutrient Deficiencies	I had some vitamin deficiencies, so would need to receive a vitamin B12 shot and up my probiotics to support my body. I would also be adding a daily dose of fermented food (sauerkraut, in my case) to my diet.

Neurotransmitters & What They're Responsible For

1. Adrenaline — This is responsible for your fight-or-flight response.
2. GABA — This helps to calm you and improve your focus levels.
3. Noradrenaline — This contracts blood vessels to increase blood flow and improve concentration.
4. Acetylcholine — This is associated with attention and learning.
5. Dopamine — This can drive feelings of pleasure or addiction.
6. Glutamine — This regulates your memory.
7. Serotonin — This is responsible for the regulation of your digestive tract and your mood. It's one of the easier neurotransmitters to hack using exercise and UV light exposure.
8. Endorphins — These heighten euphoria and reduce pain (usually during physical activity such as sex and exercise).

CHAPTER 20

Thanksgiving Rolls Around Again

Time has a funny way of escaping us, and I'm so glad that I spent the time following my diagnosis taking consistent actions to heal while focusing on gratitude and solutions rather than my problems. All of these consistent steps, no matter how small, added up to real progress. By the time Thanksgiving had rolled around again, I was feeling a bit more upbeat. This particular holiday provided the perfect time to spend the day with my children and be reminded of how endlessly thankful I am for both of them. Although I was still unable to take part in our traditional holiday hike, we enjoyed a delicious pot roast with potatoes and vegetables, followed up with some generous portions of pumpkin pie and a good movie.

The holidays have historically been the most difficult time for me to adhere to my restrictive diet. I'm still a work in progress but usually try very hard to stick to the foods that will benefit me rather than harm me. Unfortunately, when you're battling an autoimmune condition, there's no such thing as a "cheat day." Your body doesn't recognize that you just need a little break and continues to be affected by what you put in it.

Sticking to Your Guns

Sticking to a healthy regimen during the holidays is no easy feat. We're so used to being able to indulge in all the decadent treats that we've grown accustomed to that it can feel like we're missing out or depriving ourselves of a sense of normalcy. As humans, we also tend to bond over a meal. Sharing a meal with one another has been ingrained into societies around the world, and it can feel like we're not connecting as much when we're not partaking in one together. However, I need you to remind yourself that the time you get to spend and enjoy with your family is the most meaningful kind of indulgence. You can just as easily bond with them if you're not eating the same things. Once you have that mentality locked down, you can try the following:

- Eat an organic, high-protein breakfast (non-grain, non-dairy).
- Eat lots of organic vegetables and load up on filtered water throughout the day.
- Make sure you have your personal snacks with you if you're eating at someone else's house (e.g., a packet of nut butter, a gluten-free beef or turkey Chomps stick, a handful of nuts, some organic mini cucumbers, or hummus).
- Offer to come over and make an event out of cooking together so you can incorporate some of your preferred meals into the menu, or just bring over a few dishes for others to try.

CHAPTER 21

Time to Grow a New Body

"Always laugh when you can. It is cheap medicine."
~Lord Byron, 19th-century English romantic poet

The day I had been excitedly anticipating had arrived! I would be heading to Chile for the *Grow a New Body* program, hosted by Alberto and Marcelo Villoldo at their Los Lobos Lodge.

Everything about this trip brought me so much joy — even the lengthy flights it took to get there. I looked forward to my long journey on the plane, where I was free to absorb myself in the various books I had brought along and catch up on a couple shows I didn't have the chance to watch at home. Every time I have the opportunity to step into my comfy plane attire, I know I'm gearing up for an adventure!

I met the other 11 participants in my group at the airport. As we made our way to the Los Lobos Lodge, we had the chance to get to know each other a little bit. There was one woman in the group who was particularly witty and genuine, so I knew we would have fun together while healing.

We met up with our wonderful hosts and were given individual schedules that included a large variety of healing modalities. To me, this was far more exciting than hanging out at the beach on a tropical vacation. I couldn't wait to begin my personal journey. Throughout the

week, our meals were carefully planned with the purpose of putting our bodies into a state of ketosis. We were not allowed:
- Gluten
- Dairy
- Sugar
- Processed foods

We had to essentially fast between 6 p.m. and 12 p.m., with the only exceptions being tea and bone broth. Each day, we attended various appointments located around the property.

Throughout my stay in Chile, I slept in a large canvas tent with a roofless deck that allowed me to view the tranquil beauty of the moon and stars when I ventured to the bathroom during the night.

The next morning, I walked across the open field to my combined massage–chiropractic treatment, which was unlike any other massage or chiropractic treatment I had previously received. It felt as if the masseuse was tuning into my energetic field and knew exactly what my body needed. The massage was perfect and the adjustments were gentle. I typically won't let anyone touch my neck because I can't tolerate the noise or and the thought of it breaking, but I didn't even flinch this time around.

After the massage, the masseuse shared a recipe for a healthy shake as we struck up a conversation. You can try it for yourself.

Shake Recipe:
- 10-15 Brazil nuts/almonds/walnuts
- Half an avocado
- 1 banana
- ½ cup of blueberries/raspberries
- 1 scoop of maca powder
- A sprinkling of chia seeds

- 1 tbsp. of grated ginger
- 1 scoop of spirulina
- Filtered water or non-dairy milk

Footwear Freedom

After my chiropractic massage, a cranial osteopath stepped in to work on my body, instantly pinpointing the areas where energy was blocked within it. I noticeably cringed as she placed her hand on my right foot, bracing myself for the sure promise of pain. She encouraged me to relax and let her continue working, and I was amazed that I wasn't in pain while she continued applying pressure to my foot.

She felt drawn to other areas of blocked energy in my body that she seemed adept at releasing. She also noticed a lack of energy running down my right leg, so she continued to restore energy to the whole right side of my body over the course of four sessions. After working with the osteopath, I was able to put pressure on my right foot and put a shoe on for the first time in over a year! I was beside myself with joy.

I took advantage of all the healing treatments offered in the program, including:

- Acupuncture
- Glutathione IV therapy
- Oxygen therapy
- Stints in the detoxifying infrared sauna

I've found all these modalities to be beneficial to my health and would recommend looking into them to see how they could offer some relief for your own autoimmune condition.

The whole week spent in Chile revolved around a peaceful routine of mingling with the other guests, experiencing many healing methods, and enjoying delicious, healthy meals. I was fascinated by what had brought each participant to this place and cherished that special time of laughter and shared personal journeys.

One of the couples who participated in the program was grieving the devastating loss of their son, who had suffered tremendously from the same autoimmune disease I had been diagnosed with myself. Although his passing wasn't directly related to his condition, he had sadly succumbed to an unhealthy coping mechanism that had become his only source of relief from the pain. After hearing their heart-wrenching story, I suddenly became fearful and began questioning my own road to recovery.

Later that day when I went to see my host, Alberto, for my shamanic "tracking" session, I couldn't help but tear up. When I explained why I was feeling so sad and concerned, he assured me that I would be able to recover from this condition and that I needed to completely focus on my health for the next year. I had to imagine, or visualize, myself being able to run on two healthy feet.

After he tracked my energy field, Alberto informed me that I was in great health and that it was evident that I ate a nutritious diet. He saw that my autoimmune issue was not due to Karma or unhealthy living, but rather related to my father's side of the family. He explained that this was a generational issue and that this illness did not belong to me, which was a reassuring reflection of how I had personally felt about it from the start.

Alberto then said that I needed to sever that generational tie and the health-related drama attached to it — something that could be aided by a shamanic ceremony that one of the shamans would perform later that day.

The Shamans

When I met one of the shamans in her "office" in the woods, she tapped into the power of energetic healing to not only cut off the generational tie to this health crisis but to also cut the cord to my ex-husband. In her vision, she saw that my power animal was the lion, which was interesting to hear because I've always felt particularly drawn to lions. My computer screen saver at the time was an image of a lion, and I had also purchased a large metal print of a nuzzling lion and lioness to hang on my wall at home. Furthermore, she told me that I needed to embody the male energy of the lion because the male energy in my body wasn't balanced with my female energy. I had heard from several healers that the right side of the body coincides with male energy, while the left side represents the feminine energy. The shaman insisted that I needed to be strong and fearless and bold like the lion when facing decisions in my life. The lion knows that he is the king and in charge. He is agile but very strong when it's time to eat or protect.

Another shaman on-site conducted a session with me to quiet my fight-or-flight response, which can remain on overdrive even when there's no real threat, especially in those with an autoimmune condition.

Toward the end of our stay, we congregated around the bonfire and partook in a spiritual ceremony. One of our hosts sang an enchanting song, and we joined in as she circled the fire and pounded a drum. We took turns kneeling by the fire and swirling the smoke, first toward our stomachs, then our hearts, and then over our heads. We were instructed to think of the roles we wanted to release and to blow these labels into a stick we had collected earlier, tossing it into the fire thereafter. At the same time, someone stood behind us with outstretched arms for protection. It was a good reminder that while we have a variety of roles that we play throughout our lives, we are also so much more than one particular role. What is most important is our growth and evolving spirit, which can never be defined or contained.

On one of my last days in Chile, medical professionals came onsite to analyze the stool samples that we had provided. I was curious to see the results of this test since I had been taking uva ursi and berberis vulgaris to eliminate the harmful bacteria found in prior testing. The results showed that I was, in fact, healing, but Alberto said to continue the protocol and get rechecked about a month after I returned home to ensure that I was free and clear of this particular bacterium.

Upon reviewing the test results that I had brought from my naturopath at home, he also agreed that it was crucial to eliminate the high lead content in my body. He suggested taking glutathione IV injections every two weeks to help encourage the detox process.

This trip was healing on so many levels. In addition to the opportunity to try a variety of healing techniques that improved my physical health (and unearth parts of myself that had remained hidden), I also was able to forge lasting connections with other strong, resilient, spiritual people on their own healing journeys.

My favorite memories from this trip revolved around laughter. I hadn't laughed so heartily and so easily for a long time, and it was incredible how great it made me feel, both mentally and physically. Two women on this trip — one from London and one from Turkey — were particularly entertaining, and it felt phenomenal to laugh so hard that tears streamed down our cheeks. Never underestimate the healing power of laughter!

Exercise: Releasing Old Ties

Releasing old spiritual ties can be just as important as releasing old material items from your life, if not more so. If you'd like to begin releasing old ties, try the exercise below.

You will need:
- A piece of paper
- A pen or pencil
- Some sage
- A lighter
- A deep-set bowl

Now, follow the instructions:
1. Find somewhere quiet to sit.
2. On a piece of paper, write down all the negative energy, people, or ties that you want to release from your life.
3. Fold the paper up into four and say, "I release all that is not mine to carry and create space to welcome positivity and abundance into my life."
4. Light the piece of paper and drop it into the bowl.
5. Once the paper is completely burned, douse it in water and throw it out away from your home.
6. Sage your home when you get back inside and set positive intentions for your life.

This simple ritual will help you mentally and spiritually break the ties that bind you to pain and ill health.

CHAPTER 22

Holidays & Vivid Dreams

"Healing is hard. But so is constantly, desperately trying to hold yourself together."

~Samantha Camargo

Christmas Day was fast-approaching, and although I tried to add some anti-inflammatory recipes to the menu, I wasn't wholly successful, as you can see.

Christmas Day Menu
- Organic scrambled eggs, Applegate chicken sausage, and onions
- Paleo chocolate muffins
- Filet roast
- Steamed broccoli
- Stuffing
- Mashed potatoes
- Gluten-free, vegan apple pie
- See's Candies chocolate balls

Although my foot seemed to have somewhat of a reaction to some of the food, it was simply too delicious to resist. I also noticed that the eczema in my ears had flared up again, but it quickly improved as soon as I resumed my healthy eating routine. As I said before, any type of diet becomes trickier around the holidays, especially a gluten-free, dairy-free one. I will say this...it does get easier with time and practice.

My son had slipped a scratch-off lottery ticket in my stocking that year, and I won $200, so I felt confident that the Universe was still looking out for me, despite my recent indulgences.

After Christmas Day, I went to visit my friend, Hailey, and we exchanged gifts. She gave me the present that I had been looking for ever since I saw it displayed at someone's house when I last visited: a little pig with wings. To me, it represented my life and all those things that seem quite unattainable but are in fact very possible, like great health. I know that pigs will fly!

Using Your Dream Realm as a Roadmap

When people say, "follow your dreams," they probably don't mean that in the literal sense of the term. However, my dreams seemed to carry more meaning around this time, becoming increasingly vivid and frequent.

One morning, I happened to remember the details of an especially vivid dream that revolved around a man who I had met previously.

In the dream, my friend Susan and I went to an office building downtown. I saw a man from my past and his girlfriend there. At first, I pretended not to see him but then decided to approach him with a hug. It was awkward, and he didn't really return the hug. He spoke with my friend, and I overheard him say that he hadn't felt really connected to me when we were together. It really surprised me to hear this because we had so much fun together at the time. I approached him to clarify what he meant. Susan offered me an analogy by putting a few recognizable items on the table, along with a lot of little containers that didn't reveal their contents. She then said, "If you had amnesia and someone placed all these items that represent your life on the table, would you recognize yourself?" The answer to that question was "no" because not enough of myself was revealed. I told the man that my friend had offered a great analogy and that now I understood. I mentioned that someone had recently told me that I love meeting new people and having new experiences but that I take a long time to get close to people, often putting up a bit of a wall until I feel ready to reveal all of myself.

The point of this dream was that this man, as well as other people I meet, couldn't fully connect to me if I wasn't being my authentic self and sharing that with others. It's so important to be your own unique self while on this Earth. **It's everything!**

Interestingly, it was not long after this dream that I went into a new health spot in town for a smoothie and spotted Anita Moorjani's book, *Dying to Be Me: My Journey from Cancer, to Near Death, to True Healing.* If you haven't heard of Anita, she's an international speaker and New York Times best-selling author whose nearly four-year battle with cancer culminated in a near-death experience. Her book details her heavenly adventure and the lessons she learned, as well as her miraculous journey back to complete health.

I picked up the book from the shop's display shelf and randomly flipped open the page where she says, "While I was in that state of clarity in the other realm, I instinctively understood that I was dying because of all my fears. I wasn't expressing my true self because my worries were preventing me from doing so. I understood that the cancer wasn't a punishment or anything like that. It was just my own energy, manifesting as cancer because my fears weren't allowing me to express myself as the magnificent force I was meant to be." (9)

This was yet another reminder to open up and be myself!

I recommend this book if you're looking for inspiration during your own healing journey. You can find more details in the Recommended Reading & Listening section at the end of this book.

CHAPTER 23

A Costly Journey

Throughout this book, I've been very detailed in sharing my health journey with you, giving you an intimate look at the many highs and lows I've experienced along the way. This level of transparency serves a specific purpose. In addition to offering you insights, tools, and encouragement to heal, I want you to feel connected and understood, hopefully coming to the realization that if I can heal, you can too.

This brings me to the next leg of my journey.

I was determined to gain full use of my right foot again so that I could be free to walk, hike, rollerblade, and run. Most of all, I wanted to be free of all medication! A stricter diet was definitely in order.

Dr. Michael Weisman, Director of Rheumatology at Cedars-Sinai Medical Center, often speaks about the benefits of a low-starch diet and offers insights on how diet affects rheumatoid arthritis, as well as a host of other autoimmune conditions. His insights also suggested that klebsiella, a type of bacteria that feeds off starch and sugar, may have been the cause of my autoimmune condition.

I subsequently read an article about a man who went into remission from ankylosing spondylitis after adhering to a strict no-starch diet in addition to being wheat-, gluten-, and dairy-free and taking apple cider vinegar in water four times a day, all of which he cites as keys to getting better. I decided to follow his lead, trying a no-starch, no-sugar diet complete with four glasses of apple cider vinegar in water per day. Although this type of diet poses some notable challenges due to the common presence of starch and sugars in many foods, I was determined to address my chronic bloating and inflammation, with the ultimate goal of ridding myself of the pain in my foot for good.

My son commented that I had done an exceptional job of improving my health but that maybe it was time to accept my new reality. I responded that I was getting rid of this autoimmune disease and its symptoms once and for all. My goal was to be off all medication completely, and I was steadfast in my commitment to trying new possible solutions as long as the ideas kept flowing and they felt like the right thing to try instinctively.

Back to My Naturopath

By mid-January, it was time to head back to my naturopath to begin a protocol of glutathione and vitamin C IV therapy once every two weeks. I also got back the results from all my recent tests, including the heavy metal test and stool test that would reveal if the toxic levels of lead in my system had decreased and if my gut infection had resolved.

The food sensitivity test showed that I still had a high response to:
- Dairy
- Eggs
- Almonds
- Black beans
- Bananas
- Wheat and gluten

My dehydroepiandrosterone (DHEA) — a hormone naturally produced in the adrenal glands — as well as B vitamins and vitamin K were all below normal levels. The good news: my gut infection had officially bid me farewell!

I chose to avoid the foods (listed above) that my body was having a negative reaction to and take any necessary supplements to address my vitamin and DHEA deficiencies while continuing the detox protocol from my naturopath.

Bank Account Blues

If you're wondering, "How much did all of this cost?!" I wouldn't blame you. This road to self-healing can be costly. Considering that insurance doesn't cover many forms of treatment if you venture outside of the MD's office, this can be a constant concern for many. However, it's important not to get discouraged by the dollar signs. While it's likely that you'll need to dish out some cash for comprehensive testing, supplements, and unconventional treatments, remember that there are plenty of ways to better your health without breaking the bank (many of which you can find throughout this book).

Fortunately, I had some savings to fall back on when this diagnosis overtook my life, but I still needed to determine how I was going to keep myself afloat in the months to come.

I laid out all the financial possibilities in a journal while keeping an open mind, which is what I would suggest that others do too. After creating a list of five possible options to bolster my finances, I decided I would rent out my master bedroom to trade the extra living space for some money in my pocket.

You can create your own idea list with pros and cons in your journal. Start with a meditation, then write down all the creative possibilities that come to mind.

CHAPTER 24

From Appointments to Gratitude

After the appointment with my naturopath, I went back to Dr. S, who suggested that I should simplify my approach. He believed that doctors — MDs and naturopaths alike — tend to automatically throw pills at each symptom and believed that I was overcomplicating my routine. He was also well-aware that the combined cost of the various supplements and medications was quickly adding up.

Given the state of my bank account, I wholeheartedly agreed. I decided to limit my focus to the few things that would provide the most positive impact on my health. I also felt the need to work on managing my stress and relaxing my body, so Dr. S recommended yoga or Qigong as a relaxing way to remedy these issues. Qigong can enhance your mind-body connection and help return your body to its natural healing program.

Remedies All Around Me

Toward the end of January, I completed my Reiki II training and received my certification. I was now able to perform distance healings! I also indulged in a one-hour float session, which gave me the opportunity to meditate inside a giant egg-shaped pod filled with saltwater.

Once in the pod, your body temperature adjusts to that of the saltwater, becoming neither warm nor cold, while the complete silence and darkness prompts a state of total sensory deprivation. If you aren't particularly claustrophobic, a float pod session can offer many benefits:

- Stress reduction
- Anxiety relief
- Pain relief
- Relaxation
- Headache reduction
- Increase in circulation
- Restful sleep

The major bonus: absolute peace!

Gratitude from Pain

Around this same time, I noticed that my foot had been more swollen over the course of a week, and I was desperate to pinpoint the cause. In my mind, there were only two possible culprits: something I was eating or the fact that I only had a couple of months to financially make it or break it. I was well-aware that stress and an unhealthy diet tend to team up to contribute to the flare-up of autoimmune symptoms. Despite my discomfort, I was still able to jot down a gratitude list on this day. Have a look at it as a source of inspiration for your own.

- My dog, Lucy, curled up sweetly next to me.
- My children, who I love so much! They are both so creative and talented, and I believe they are both on this Earth to positively influence the lives of many people in this world.
- Northern California weather — both the rain and the sunshine.
- Great friendships — old and new!
- My loving and supportive family that makes me laugh. I love that we all keep learning and growing together.
- My comfortable bed and my whole house, which feels so inviting and cozy.
- My tenant, who contributes financially…and is also a fantastic person and friend.

- The journey of healing I've been on this past year, discovering healing solutions and meeting phenomenal people in the process.
- The kindness of strangers, especially while I was on crutches.
- Interesting literature — I have found many great books to inspire or educate myself.
- My meditations, which bring me peace and creative solutions.
- Tests that help me learn more about my health.
- My resilience, tenacity, and creativity, which I can apply toward finding optimal health.
- Faith in God/the Universe and my own intuition.
- Having a vehicle that takes me to my next great adventure…or just to the store for a snack.

I believe it's quite valuable to create a gratitude list whenever you start to feel stressed or less hopeful. This will create a positive energy shift.

CHAPTER 25

Inspiration is All Around You

Part of the process of developing your gratitude and healing is understanding that you're not alone on your journey. There are countless people just like us who grapple with autoimmune conditions, sometimes taking years to get a proper diagnosis. Yolanda Hadid, a former model and TV personality, struggled publicly with Lyme disease. She has posted on Instagram quite avidly, detailing her Lyme journey, and written a book about her recovery titled *Believe Me*. As I scrolled through Yolanda's Instagram account, I noticed a comment from a woman who had discovered that her 20-year struggle with fibromyalgia was really a misdiagnosed case of Lyme disease. Furthermore, the Lyme testing that she had done through Labcorp and Quest was negative, but the testing done through the IGeneX Lab in California showed a positive result for Borrelia burgdorferi. She stated that it was so worth it because she is now on a very different path and finally has hope for a healthy future.

I had also heard that many people with rheumatoid arthritis actually have Lyme, so it was definitely something worth ruling out.

Symptoms of Lyme Disease

Lyme disease can masquerade as an autoimmune disease, so be on the lookout for the following symptoms that may go undetected:

- Fever
- Headache

- Fatigue
- A skin rash called erythema migrans

If left untreated, prolonged symptoms can include:
- Severe headaches
- Neck stiffness
- Unexplained rashes around the body
- Droopiness on one or both sides of the face (palsy)
- Severe joint aches, swelling, and arthritis
- Muscular, tendon, bone, and joint pain
- Irregular heartbeat or palpitations
- Dizzy spells
- Shortness of breath
- Nerve pain
- Tingling sensations and shooting pain in the hands or feet
- Eventual inflammation of the spinal cord and brain

If you have any of these symptoms, it's important to get yourself tested for Lyme through a reputable, specialized testing center.

As February approached, my foot seemed less swollen. I began to see a definite link between the food that I ate and my condition. I continued with my vitamin C and glutathione IV therapy.

More inspiration came my way in the form of something unexpected. I meditated one day, centering my focus on creating a thriving business and discovering the various ways that I could bring money into my home. The very next day, I received a Venmo notice. A woman, to whom I had loaned $500 two years prior, had paid me back what she owed plus interest. I honestly hadn't expected to get the money back, so this was a nice surprise. It also solidified my belief that meditation is a powerful tool to cultivate what you desire.

CHAPTER 26

GUT HEALTH & TAPPING

In the first week of February 2017, I received a book that I had ordered titled *Living A.S. Free* by Micah Cranman. The book details the story of a man who overcame his ankylosing spondylitis symptoms mainly through diet. A special cookbook was included, which featured recipes to help combat this particular autoimmune condition. Something that stood out to me was Micah's reasoning for why he would never take methotrexate to treat his symptoms:

- The negative side effects
- How the drug compromises the body's ability to produce DNA
- How the drug prevents the cells of the gastrointestinal tract from dividing rapidly enough to stay healthy

The Disease-Modifying Antirheumatic Drug (DMARD) that he found success with is sulfasalazine, a common treatment for Crohn's disease that lowers inflammation in the gut and intestinal tract without further damaging the gut or suppressing the immune system. It allows the gut to heal, thereby preventing klebsiella and other toxins from leaking out and causing an immune response. This drug is designed to treat the root cause of A.S. (inflamed leaky gut) rather than just the symptoms.

He states that an enteric-coated version should be used, as more of the drug will be delivered where the anti-inflammatory effects are most important, in the lower intestine.

To continue healing my gut, I kept on my daily regimen of:
- Apple cider vinegar with water
- 1 tbsp. of coconut oil in bone broth
- A small dish of prebiotic sauerkraut

I made it a point to switch out my body lotions in exchange for organic coconut oil, wanting to avoid unknown chemicals at all costs. Additionally, I had begun doing a small workout routine involving:
- Squats with a kettlebell
- 10 lb weights for arm strengthening
- Light stretching after each workout

Find a workout that works for you: one that's tailored to your symptoms or potential mobility issues. YouTube is a fantastic place to find a variety of workouts, and you're likely to find at least one or two that are specifically suited to you.

EFT Tapping

Around this time, I delved into the world of Emotional Freedom Technique (EFT) tapping. Designed to help with a wide range of emotional and physical ailments, such as stress, anxiety, and even pain, this method involves tapping specific acupressure points on your body while focusing on an emotion, experience, or issue you want to release.

According to Nick Ortner, author of the New York Times best-selling book, *The Tapping Solution: A Revolutionary System for Stress-Free Living*:

"There's nothing wrong with venting, letting off a little steam. The problem comes when you find yourself venting about the same thing repeatedly, with no change and no resolution. Add tapping to the venting and a few things will happen. You'll let go of the story much faster. b. You'll begin to come to a new awareness about the issue. c. You'll naturally come up with creative solutions. I've had many people tell me that there's no solution to a particular situation. I nod and ask them to tap while telling me about their stress, or anger, or sadness. More often than not, they discover potential solutions they didn't even believe existed, right there in real time." (10)

With my curiosity piqued, I tuned in to a recording from Nick Ortner himself, following along as he described how to conduct the tapping routine three times in a row.

After completing this simple healing method, I got out of bed and was able to put full pressure on my right foot. I was even able to walk around without a limp!

It brought tears to my eyes because I truly hadn't felt the bottom of my foot in a very long time due to the inflammation. Given the fact that the sensation lasted half the day, tapping is something that I would recommend you try.

Exercise: Tapping Techniques

1. First, think of the problem you want to resolve. It's important to only focus on one problem at a time.
2. Next, rank the problem so that you can analyze how successful the tapping has been at the end of it. On a scale of 1-10, is this the worst the problem has ever been?
3. Set yourself up for acceptance. You can say: "Despite having this [specific problem], I am completely accepting of myself in this moment." This is the phrase you'll want to hold on to as you begin tapping.
4. Continue repeating the phrase as you begin tapping on your body with the tips of your fingers. Follow this sequence:
    a. The top of your head, directly in the center;

    b. The starting point of your eyebrows, near your nose;
    c. The outer corner of your eye, on the bone;
    d. Under your eye, on the bone;
    e. Under your nose, in the center of your nose and upper lip;
    f. Your chin, between the base of your jaw and your lower lip;
    g. The center or beginning of your collarbone;
    h. The side of your upper abdomen; just below the armpit.
5. Tap on each point five times before moving on.
6. Now, rate the severity of the problem again — once the tapping is done.

Some of you might experience positive changes immediately, as I did, but for others, it may take time. Keep at it for a few days or move on to something that suits you better.

CHAPTER 27

ADVOCATING FOR THE RIGHT TREATMENTS

"Ordinary people believe only in the possible. Extraordinary people visualize not what is possible or probable, but rather what is impossible. And by visualizing the impossible, they begin to see it as possible."

~Cherie Carter-Scott

In February, I went back to see Dr. S, informing him that I wanted to forgo the methotrexate in exchange for sulfasalazine in order to heal my gut without suppressing my immune system or compromising my body's ability to produce DNA. Following his go-ahead, I picked up my new prescription, which the pharmacist said is also used for anxiety and depression, and began my new regimen of taking two pills, twice a day.

Shortly after I began taking the medication, I ironically began to feel a bit anxious. However, my foot still seemed to be faring well since switching medications. It looked a little red but didn't feel particularly hot, cold, or more inflamed than usual. The redness I noticed may have coincided with the increased circulation in my right foot, which was a positive outcome. It was at this point that I watched the Autoimmune Revolution Q&A online. Hosted by Dr. Peter Osborne, author of *No Grain, No Pain*, the discussion focused on why one may not be healing from an autoimmune condition. He mentioned that if you aren't getting better, you should check the "Big 4" below:

1. Bacterial gut infections
2. Food intolerances
3. Heavy metals
4. Vitamin/mineral deficiencies

I ticked all the boxes. If you do as well, it's essential that you work on these four elements to speed up the process of healing.

As per Dr. Osborne's discussion points, I encourage you to check your food and supplement labels to avoid consuming all sources of gluten and all grains (including quinoa). You can also get genetically tested for gluten intolerance. This type of test can be found on the Gluten Free Society website. It's imperative to work with a doctor who understands gluten the same way that Dr. Osborne does, so keep that in mind when searching for a naturopath or functional medicine doctor in your area.

When you're coping with the consequences of a health issue, it can be easy to become somewhat of a recluse and stop doing the activities you once enjoyed. Meeting up with friends for dinner or drinks becomes less entertaining when you're on such a strict diet. Not being able to physically do the job or engage in the hobby you used to enjoy quickly becomes frustrating.

I've always liked to have adventure in my life, as well as a sense of connection with other people. In the months following my diagnosis, I needed to essentially reinvent myself by coming up with new interests that would bring me that same sense of connection and excitement.

Luckily, I've found yoga to be a great activity for relaxing and stretching, as well as quieting the mind, so I decided to take advantage of a special deal at a yoga studio nearby. For one reasonable price, I could take as many classes as I wanted for three weeks. I ended up going daily and trying various types of yoga. At the end of the three weeks, I found that I was more limber and felt better overall. You may consider incorporating a form of resistance training to improve muscle strength, reduce stress on your joints, and support immune regulation.

I also realized that I needed a mental break, so I met up with a friend. Our activities included shopping, having a healthy lunch, and making a trip to Barnes & Noble, one of my favorite destinations. Inspiration came to me while reading books by Mike Dooley, Dr. Joe Dispenza, and Gregg Braden. All three authors speak about creating your reality with the power of your thoughts, emphasizing that you should back those thoughts up with emotion.

I believe that philosophy so wholeheartedly because I've experienced it. Even after how far I had come on my healing journey, I still needed to remind myself to focus on those things I wanted in my life. I had to be disciplined in doing that more often and truly feeling it on an emotional level. Understand that you'll have moments when you stray off course. This is only natural. You must make a conscious effort to recenter yourself.

My Visualizations in February
- I will visualize myself walking into various doctors' offices and having them be so surprised by my complete recovery, as evidenced by my improved blood work and overall condition, despite the elimination of prednisone and methotrexate.
- I will imagine writing a book about my healing journey that will help others avoid unnecessary pain.
- I will imagine my finances coming together in amazing ways through great renters and more photography clients. I will create extra income doing something I enjoy.

- Things have worked out perfectly in the past, and this visualization list will be no exception.
- Lastly, I will imagine lacing up a pair of roller skates and zooming around the roller rink once again!

Keep putting your intentions out into the Universe and patiently wait to be pleasantly surprised.

Visualization Exercise!

Take a moment to create your own visualization list, including at least five items that would make you happy if you were to accomplish them.

CHAPTER 28

A Wake-up Call to Go Grain-Free

"What we see mainly depends on what we look for."
~John Lubbock

By February 21, I was growing increasingly concerned with my financial situation. My major concern was that if my photography business didn't take off within the next month, I would be in a real pickle. I didn't want to feel rushed into selling my home, especially when I didn't have another destination in mind, and the thought of it was becoming increasingly stressful. I spoke with my mom and relayed my financial concerns.

Reaching out to someone who knows you best in situations like these can be a lifeline. My mom reminded me that I have always been able to think positively and that my life has always come together. It was a comforting reminder that I shouldn't make any decisions when I am in "fear mode" and that when I imagine positive outcomes, I will produce them.

Fear Mode Decisions

Fear throws everything out of whack. When you try to make decisions in a fearful or anxious state, odds are you won't make the right ones. This can be chalked up to the fact that fear interferes with emotional regulation, which is vital in any sound decision-making process. You're more

likely to make impulsive decisions based on your fear rather than on your actual reality. To prevent yourself from making decisions out of fear:
- Take a moment to sit quietly and reflect, tuning in to how your body feels as you imagine each of the choices you're contemplating. Give yourself a few days to mull things over if this is going to be a life-changing decision.
- Write down the pros and cons of the decision you're about to make.
- Ask yourself if this aligns with the vision you have for your life.
- If not, are there any alternative options?

While I was still benefiting from my vitamin C and glutathione IV therapy sessions, I found myself veering off track in late February. I consumed everything that I shouldn't have, including:
- Garlic truffle fries
- Champagne
- Gluten-free chocolate tiramisu (dairy included)
- Flourless chocolate cupcakes

My foot became noticeably red, which was no surprise after my food rebellion. When you've tried so many methods of healing but just aren't positive if you'll finally crack the optimal health code…well…you rebel a little.

NOTE: While it's not advised, sometimes you just need to re-experience that bit of discomfort for yourself. When you rebel against your new diet or lifestyle and suffer the repercussions, it reaffirms the notion that you should stick to what you're doing. It's working, so keep going!

Back On Track

As they say, it's not how many times you fall but how many times you get back up. That's what matters the most.

In March of 2017, I made a conscious decision to get back on track and commit to Dr. Peter Osborne's 30-Day Gluten Free Challenge, listed in *No Grain, No Pain*. Day 1 was intense with my foot being a bit swollen. However, my back didn't cramp up and bother me as it had the day before. On Day 2 of the challenge, I was inspired to make a few of the recipes in the book to see if they could eliminate my symptoms, and they did seem to help!

My mood continued to improve, and I believed that the new grain-free diet was helpful in this regard. In addition, I found alternative solutions to my financial predicament. During meditation, I came up with the idea of becoming a Lyft driver, which would provide extra income and offer me a flexible schedule, as well as allow me to be off my feet. If you have a vehicle and a flexible schedule, driving for a service like Lyft or Uber could be a viable option for side income.

CHAPTER 29

A Toothy Grin

My teeth had been troubling me. I was struggling with sensitivity in a few different areas, so I decided to make another visit to my dentist. One thing he suggested was wearing a mouthguard at night to prevent any further damage from grinding my teeth. The pressure tends to create small fractures in the tooth, which sensitizes the tooth and creates a breeding ground for bacteria.

Symptoms of Bruxism

When we're in pain or dealing with trauma, it's quite common to grind our teeth (a condition known as "bruxism"). Most of us will grind our teeth at night, as this is the time when our bodies go through involuntary motions that are tied to our subconscious feelings. If you have any of the following symptoms, it might be worth a trip to your dentist:

- Facial pain
- Neck and shoulder pain
- A tense, painful, or stiff jaw
- Worn-down, chipped, or broken teeth
- Increased tooth sensitivity
- Headaches
- Sleep disturbances
- Earache

If you are diagnosed with bruxism, try some calming meditations before bed. You can also journal about everything that has been bothering you, followed up by everything you were grateful for that day. Tell yourself that tomorrow is a new day and that you will not be carrying today's stress into dreamland with you. Also, wear a mouthguard if you're prescribed one.

My dentist and I discussed my root canal as well as the research of Dr. Dietrich Klinghardt, a doctor in applied medical neurobiology and the founder of the Sophia Health Institute.

His research states that most root canals are infected and can also be the cause of, or worsen, some autoimmune symptoms. The dentist wasn't completely convinced but was willing to let me use his 3D X-ray machine to determine what was going on in my mouth. The X-ray revealed a small infection at the base of my root canal. He believed the infection was quite minor and not something that would have shown up without this special 3D machine but that he would go over the option of replacing the root canal with an implant if that's what I wanted to do. I knew he didn't think that my root canal had any effect on my health issues, but I needed to address every possibility for the sake of improving my condition.

The morning after my visit to the dentist, I woke up and found the Natural Health 365 oral health podcast in my email. It revolved around how the cause of your illness may stem from issues in your mouth, such as infections from root canals, mercury fillings, and incompatible materials. There is blood work that can be done — known as a biocompatibility test — to show which dental materials are incompatible with your body. This specific test can be ordered through Biocomp Laboratories. The timing was interesting since I had just inquired about this type of information at my last trip to the dentist. It seemed as if another synchronicity was steadily urging me along my path.

At this point, I was very interested in taking the biocompatibility test that was suggested and continuing my quest for optimal health. I felt so incredibly close to completely resolving my symptoms and, subsequently, being able to help other family members, friends, and strangers with their health as well.

CHAPTER 30

Taxi Talks & Tucson

The synchronicities continued as my next Lyft passenger happened to be just as interested in healing modalities as I was. Somewhere along the drive, we arrived at the topic of infrared saunas, and I was amazed to find out that he had his own infrared sauna at home.

I truly believe that we draw people to us who are operating at the same vibrational level as we are, or that we are put in each other's path for a reason. When I think back to my very first passenger, I'm reminded that you cannot judge or know who a person is based on their appearance. I always meet interesting, fun people and continually learn from them.

The aforementioned passenger was a young, large, Hispanic man with various tattoos across his body. We struck up a conversation as I drove him to the airport, during which I discovered he was on his own spiritual journey and was headed to stay with shamans for a month. This, again, reinforced the idea that your energy draws in similar energy.

My second passenger was a man from India who worked in the fashion industry and had a great outlook on life. He seemed to truly know how to live in the moment and appreciate life. He even said that he asks for some difficult moments so that he is always sure to truly appreciate the great ones.

Easter Excitement

I was excited about my next adventure: another trip to Arizona! I would be visiting my family in Tucson for Easter.

A trip to Tucson is always something I look forward too. Everyone in my family has a creative side, so it's always fun to work on various projects together. Whether it involves photography, art, theater, or product creation, we always seem to have the best time. This is the only group of people that I feel I can completely be myself around, without censoring any part of myself. We can also discuss spirituality and many other topics with an open mind, and new ideas are viewed as innovative or interesting, rather than crazy. If you don't have this type of family support, especially as you fight to recover from a serious illness, I would suggest finding a supportive community amongst friends or with a particular meetup group that covers a topic you're drawn to. You can also look into Facebook groups and free webinars around your condition that allow you to mingle online afterward.

While in Arizona, I was able to tag along with my brother to his first appointment with a local naturopath. I had been encouraging him to take aggressive measures regarding his own health, and after 30 years of living with Crohn's, various medications, and multiple surgeries, he was ready to try something new. I hope some of you, who might have lived with your condition for decades and who are reading this right now, know that there is no deadline for recovery. **You can start right now, where you are, with what you have, and commit to becoming a healthier version of yourself.**

Inspiration struck me in Tucson, and I started defining what I wanted to include in my book on healing – yes, this very book! I also began detailing how I would plan a transformative retreat for women that would center around the theme of teaching them how to live outside of their comfort zones and embrace their authentic selves.

I returned home with this newfound energy coursing through my veins.

CHAPTER 31

Keep Testing

"Genetics load the gun, environment pulls the trigger."
~Francis Collins

Again, I need to stress the importance of continual testing. Your results will tell you if your health regimen is working or if it isn't and, quite possibly, what you need to change. In this chapter, I'm going to walk you through some of the test results that continued coming in from March of 2017 through May of that same year. Hopefully, these will offer you some insight into what worked for me and therefore what might work for you, as well as the specific tests that you might need to take.

In March, my stool test showed no further signs of infection, also revealing that the toxic overload shown in past tests had diminished. What I really needed to find out was whether I was detoxing the heavy metals and other toxins sufficiently.

MTHFR Gene

Methylenetetrahydrofolate reductase (MTHFR) is a gene and enzyme that helps to process the folate we eat into a nutrient our bodies can utilize. People who have MTHFR mutations have an interruption in the "methylation pathway." Methylation affects more than 20 different processes in our bodies, including regulating gene expression, and when interrupted, can disrupt many essential bodily functions. If you have this particular mutation, your doctor can suggest alternative ways to ensure you're getting the proper nutrients you need.

The two most-studied mutations of this MTHFR gene (C677T and A1298C) are linked to a host of chronic health conditions. These mutations impact homocysteine levels in the blood, which can be associated with the lowered ability to detoxify and a risk factor for cardiovascular disease. They can also influence sensitivity to and dosing requirements of methotrexate.

I got tested for these mutations by taking the MTHFR genotype test, which you can schedule through your naturopath or functional medicine doctor. My test results showed that I was positive for the C677T mutation and negative for the A1298C mutation. This indicated that my enzyme activity was about 60% normal but didn't correlate with increased homocysteine levels, increased risk of cardiovascular disease or thrombosis, or methotrexate intolerance or lower dose requirements.

People with impaired MTHFR genetic functioning may have to be especially careful of the toxins they come into contact with because their bodies struggle to eliminate them. This means that filtering drinking water (known to contain arsenic and other toxins) by installing filters on taps and showerheads is important. Additionally, cutting out toxic beauty products and personal care items will also reduce the burden put on your MTHFR enzyme.

Knowledge Is Power

According to Dr. Amy Myers, there are six ways to overcome MTHFR mutations:
1. Supplement with pre-methylated B vitamins.
2. Avoid folic acid (synthetic B vitamins) because your body is unable to convert it.

3. Eat foods rich in B vitamins.
4. Reduce your toxic burden: filter air and water, remove amalgam dental fillings safely, and avoid fish containing high levels of mercury.
5. Flush out toxins safely by supporting detox pathways.
6. Balance your MTHFR mutation with supplements (including glutathione, liver support, and magnesium) to support detoxification. (11)

Test Results & Possibilities

In April, I had a phone consultation with Dr. Osborne from Origins Healthcare to go over all my test results, including those from my naturopath. These were the results.

Test	Result
ELISA/ACT LRA (identifies delayed immune responses to food and chemicals)	STRONG reactions to: Onion (yellow), FD&C Green #3, Red Chili Pepper, Glyphosate, and Propyl Gallate MODERATE reactions to: Lemon, Red Leaf Lettuce, Mercury, Honey, Okra, FD&C Red #40, Rhodotorula, Tert-Butyl-Methyl Ether (TBME), Yogurt (Cow), Acai Berry, and Cis-Dichloroethylene (1,2-Dichloroethylene)

I'm glad that I had this more in-depth allergy testing done because it gave me so much insight into what I should avoid. I knew to stop eating yellow onions, which had ironically been a regular part of my diet since my healing journey began, and eat only locally grown, organic foods to avoid the glyphosate found in "Roundup," an herbicide sprayed on crops to deter pests. I also checked my food, toothpaste, and mouthwash for propyl gallate, tossing anything that listed it in its ingredients. Ask your doctor for additional information about avoiding and detoxing this preservative from your body.

TBME is a chemical compound found in air and water as a result of fuel exhaust fumes. Dr. Osborne advised me to use my car's "recirculate air" setting while driving on the highway. That would keep external air — and the unwanted chemicals that came with it — out of my car in favor of the clean air recirculating in the cabin, especially while idling in traffic amidst all those exhaust fumes.

Rhodotorula is a type of mold that falls on the natural yeast side of the spectrum. It can be found in soil, air, the ocean, lakes, water, certain fruit juices, and milk. If you're interested in having your home tested for mold, you might start with a simple test kit through a website like gotmold.com or one you find based on your own research.

The FD&C dyes are found in food, drugs, and cosmetics, so it's important to read the ingredients on every label.

The Cis-Dichloroethylene can be found in your water and in over-the-counter fish oils. It can also be found in decaf coffee and tea as a result of being imparted on the coffee or tea during the process of removing the caffeine. Make sure your water at home is filtered, and opt for organic, herbal teas.

Dr. Osborn instructed me to avoid all strongly reactive foods for eight months while eliminating the moderately reactive foods for six months. I was also told not to reintroduce foods from either category back into my diet until we had a follow-up conversation.

If you have similar symptoms to my own and would like to find out whether certain foods might be having an effect on you, it's always advisable to have the proper testing done.

Test	Result
OMEGA CHECK REPORT	EPA and DHA levels would need to be raised. These particular omega-3 fatty acids support brain and heart health and help regulate cell inflammation (among other things).

You can increase your EPA and DHA by eating cold-water fish like salmon, sardines, and mackerel. My omega-6/omega-3 ratio was also off, which was even more reason for me to indulge in cold-water fish, as well as others foods high in omega-3s, like flaxseeds and walnuts. To reduce the omega-6s, I needed to limit processed foods and vegetable oils.

Omega-3s and omega-6s are both fatty acids essential to our health. However, with our modern Western diet, we tend to ingest more omega-6s and disturb the correct balance between the two. In addition, the omega-6s we ingest tend to be damaged by their exposure to oxygen or heat, leading to negative health effects.

Test	Result
QUEST TEST FOR IRON AND FERRITIN	Iron and ferritin were low.

According to Quest Diagnostics, your iron levels should be 50-170 mcg/dL for women. Mine was 68. Your ferritin levels should be 13-150 ng/mL, and mine was 19. This was an improvement from when I tested my ferritin level back in 2015 and discovered it was a 4!

Test	Result
HEAVY METAL TEST	The report stated: This individual's lead exceeds three times the upper expected limit per the reference population. Because a percentage of absorbed or assimilated lead is excreted in urine, the urine lead level reflects recent or ongoing exposure to lead and the degree of excretion or detoxification.

This test result was rather concerning, but it did mention that the lead levels could be reflective of the degree of detoxification. I began to wonder if all the detoxing I had been doing had been pulling long-stored lead out of my bones and tissues and into my blood, where it is generally more recognizable.

Regardless of where it was coming from, I knew I needed to get it out of my system as soon as possible. I had been carrying on with the vitamin C and glutathione IV therapy for six months and taking HM Chelate and liver support to assist the detox process. The following are the questions that sprang to mind, some of which you might want to relay to your practitioner if you find yourself in this position:

- Am I pulling so much lead out of my bones and brain tissue that it's now only visible in the bloodstream, and thus, the test?
- Do I have enough binders in place to prevent the lead from getting reabsorbed in my body?
- Am I continually being exposed to lead by a source that I'm unaware of?

Test	Result
QUEST VITAMIN D,25-OH TEST PANEL	My vitamin D level was 72 ng/mL.

When you have an autoimmune condition, the therapeutic level is 50-80 ng/mL. I was definitely in the correct range.

Test	Result
SPECTRACELL NUTRITIONAL DEFICIENCY TEST	I was functionally deficient in serine and glutamine. I had 15 borderline deficiencies, which included B vitamins (B1, B2, B3, B6, B12).

B vitamin deficiencies seem to go hand in hand with autoimmune conditions. Dr. Osborne recommended taking L-serine and glutamine supplements. I didn't need to add extra supplementation for the borderline deficiencies.

Test	Result
COMPREHENSIVE DRINKING WATER ANALYSIS	The test showed there were no "unacceptable" levels of any primary metals, secondary metals, or fluoride. The pH balance showed a level of 7.6, which was also acceptable.

I ran the Comprehensive Drinking Water Analysis test on my own to reassure myself that my water filtration system at home was working properly. pH levels below 7 are considered acidic, while pH levels above 7 are considered alkaline. A pH level of 7 is neutral, being neither acidic nor alkaline.

It certainly was a lot to take in all at once, but I was more motivated than ever to remedy these issues. I ordered the supplements Dr. Osborne recommended through Origins Healthcare Center, feeling especially inclined to order my supplements through this particular center because of their commitment to high-quality and gluten-free ingredients. Dr. Osborne advised me to forgo the prescription folic acid I had been taking since I wasn't deficient in it. Moreover, it includes dyes for the green and yellow color, which can pose health risks.

Regarding my root canal, Dr. Osborne suggested testing for the type of infection and considering replacing the tooth with an implant made from materials that I wasn't sensitive to. If you were to just remove the tooth, the tooth above it would deteriorate due to the lack of pressure from the opposing tooth. The teeth beside the gap might also shift and become misaligned. Furthermore, the location of this particular tooth was very noticeable, so I didn't want to have it pulled without the option of a quick replacement.

CHAPTER 32

Could It be Toxic Mold?

In May of 2017, I tried a full-spectrum CBD tincture that was meant to alleviate the pain and pressure in my foot. It did decrease some of the inflammation, serving as another sure sign of how important it is to be open to medicinal herbs, tinctures, and remedies that fall outside the spectrum of traditional or Western medicine.

By June, my levels of mental and physical exhaustion had begun to take a toll. One day, I accidentally dozed off during an afternoon meditation session and didn't wake up for four whole hours! I assumed that my iron deficiency may have been rearing its ugly head once again, but I also questioned whether any undetected mold in my home may have been the true culprit. I thought back to the previous leaks under my refrigerator and bathroom sink and wondered if any toxic mold was lingering where the eye couldn't see, well-aware of the fact that this sneaky saboteur could trigger disease and hinder healing.

The following month, I decided to do something about my suspicions, scheduling two mold companies to come out to inspect my home. Neither of the professionals from the two companies could see or smell any potential mold. One suggested that I do an air test to pinpoint exactly where the mold might be hiding. As much as I hated to spend more money on testing, I also didn't want to be living with toxic mold and having it affect my recovery. The result of the air test showed no issue with mold, so I checked that off my list and started a different heavy metal detox protocol through Dr. Osborne, in hopes that it would alleviate some of my lingering symptoms. I used ethylenediaminetetraacetic acid (EDTA), taking it in sequences of three days on and then 11 days off. I did this continuously for four months.

CHAPTER 33

Healing Strides and Tiny Miracles

By October 3, I had a reason to celebrate: I was finally off all the medications the doctor had prescribed! I was thrilled to know that all my less-than-conventional efforts to heal were paying off. Throughout the following two months, I added one dropperful of the CBD tincture to my daily routine and occasionally rubbed Frankincense oil on my toe joints and the ball of my foot.

While this self-treatment seemed to reduce the inflammation in my foot intermittently, most mornings delivered the familiar discomfort of trying to walk barefoot.

On the evening of November 26 (two years from the day that I first became dependent on crutches), I felt a noticeable difference in my foot as I made dinner. It seemed less inflamed, so I tested it out by taking my shoe off and walking directly on it. I was amazed to discover that my foot felt completely fine! I could actually **feel** my entire foot touching the floor, this time without the inflammation dulling the sensation. I had to push the boundaries to see how far I could take this newfound mobility, so I jogged across the kitchen floor. Again, I felt no pain or discomfort. The final test was seeing if I could put on a closed-toed shoe and run. I can't tell you how beside myself with awe I was when I could get a closed-toe shoe on my foot. It was time to venture outside to find a more open space to run further and faster. I found what little light I could under the streetlamp and had my son take a video of me as I began a steady jog down the street.

I COULD RUN!

I was too excited to wait until the light of day to share this with everyone who had been supporting me throughout this health journey, so I immediately posted the news on my Facebook page. This was a major step — pun totally intended — toward optimal health and healing! I wanted to share my fabulous news with as many people as possible, as quickly as I could.

I was RUNNING in a CLOSED-TOED SHOE!

I was off all the medications that the doctors had prescribed and was now able to run! The comments and texts started rolling in as friends began asking me what I had done differently that day. What had I done that would allow me to run for the first time in **two years**? I will say that, even though I had taken some CBD oil and applied frankincense oil to my foot a couple nights prior, my success could be credited to my cumulative efforts to unburden my immune system, one layer at a time, through diet, supplementation, detoxification of heavy metals, stress management, and gut infection healing.

Going Infrared

Shortly after the night of my miraculous run down the street, I splurged and bought myself the infrared sauna I had been eyeing for months. I was well-aware of the healing benefits of this type of spa thanks to past research and my transformative stay in Chile. What pushed me to finally get one of my own? Well, I had been listening to The Green Smoothie Girl online, who had expanded on the benefits further. She spoke of a particular company that was offering a limited-time discount on their spas during the holidays. I had been wanting to purchase one of my own for quite some time — in fact, since I had ordered my infrared healing mat — and I couldn't pass up this special (and synchronistic!) deal.

The infrared sauna turned out to be the best Christmas gift I could have given myself. The company that makes this particular sauna uses cedar, which won't mold, and notably avoids toxic wood stains, glues, and chemicals in the construction process. The sauna also emits the lowest electromagnetic fields (EMFs) in comparison to other saunas in its class, such as those created by other commercial spa companies.

With my new spa set up on the back patio, I now had an additional detox tool at my disposal.

Benefits of Infrared Saunas

If you'd like to purchase your own infrared sauna and have the finances to do so, I believe it's worth it. The benefits include:
- Encouraging the widening of blood vessels and increased blood flow, thus supporting heart health
- Improving blood circulation, which soothes aching muscles
- Reducing severe or chronic pain
- Assisting with detoxification
- Reducing inflammation
- Relaxing your body and reducing oxidative stress, which, in turn, boosts your health
- Promoting better sleep

NOTE: Remember to stay well-hydrated while using the sauna (I like to bring 16-32 ounces of ice water with me). Remove yourself right away if you start to feel dizzy or nauseous. Also, shower immediately after you exit the sauna to wash away the toxins you eliminated before they get reabsorbed into your body. Check with your own doctor before using the infrared sauna if you have preexisting conditions that might be affected negatively by the heat.

Overall, the sauna was a worthy splurge, as it now provides me with added healing, detoxifying, and pain-relieving power.

CHAPTER 34

Minerals, Nutrients, & Parasites

January 2018 — It had now been a bit over two years since I had first experienced that ominous pain in my foot. At this stage, I had been detoxing heavy metals with the aid of my infrared sauna every other day. I had also been incorporating coffee enemas on those same days to aid the detoxification process. In case you haven't heard of a coffee enema yet, let me tell you why you might want to check into it.

Coffee Enemas

Coffee enemas offer some distinct differences in comparison to standard water enemas. While water enemas clean out your colon, the major benefit of coffee enemas is liver detoxification. The coffee stimulates your liver to release, and then recirculate, the bile where toxins are stored. By releasing these toxins, it allows the liver to start removing additional toxins from your body. Furthermore, according to a paper published in the National Library of Medicine, "The kahweol and cafestol in coffee enhance the activity of glutathione (GSH) S-transferase (GST), a major antioxidant enzyme that neutralizes free radicals by 600% to 700%." (12) This has even been known to assist in the treatment of certain cancers.

Every time I completed a coffee enema, any lingering swelling in my foot would disappear, so I knew it was effective. I also felt clearer-headed and focused, and I was able to get more things accomplished throughout the day.

It was important to replenish any minerals in my body that the sauna and enemas might have depleted by taking a daily trace mineral supplement. I also drank a tall glass of water with chlorophyll drops 30 minutes before each enema to ensure that the toxins were properly bound and carried out of my system. I took another dose of the chlorophyll in water 30 minutes before my next meal (after the enema) because research has shown that more toxins will be dumped into your system at this time.

Parasites & Heavy Metals

In January of 2018, my micronutrient panel revealed that I was still deficient in a number of vitamins and minerals, including B vitamins. Parasites seemed like a plausible reason for why I didn't seem to be absorbing the nutrients from my food and continued to be deficient in many vitamins and minerals.

After watching a Parasite and Heavy Metal Summit online, I learned that you must address the parasites in your body, as well as heavy metals, if you want to regain your health completely. Certain parasites feed off the heavy metals in your body, acting as their hosts. Therefore, if you want to rid yourself of heavy metals, you'll need to eliminate all the parasites that are keeping them trapped in their bodies and, therefore, trapped in your own body. With this in mind, I ordered the Foundational Protocol from CellCore Biosciences, which consisted of anti-parasite support capsules that I took consistently throughout the day. It was simple but quite effective, in my opinion.

Dr. Klinghardt was one of the expert speakers at the Parasite and Heavy Metal Summit. It just so happens that he was also one of the doctors that helped former model and TV personality Yolanda Hadid regain her health after being hit hard by Lyme disease. During the summit, he mentioned that although there is no comprehensive testing method available for parasites, many people have them. While most standard tests can only detect a limited number of specific parasites (without taking the larger population of parasites into account), he personally uses the Autonomic Response Testing (A.R.T.) protocol he developed, which utilizes muscle biofeedback with great results. However, the easiest way to confirm the potential presence of parasites on your own is to simply start the parasite cleanse and take a quick peek into the toilet. You'll know within a very short period whether you have them or not because they'll start appearing in your stool.

On the fourth day of my CellCore parasite cleanse, upon wiping, I felt something somewhat rubbery in the waste. Later in the week, I discovered what looked like a very long rope worm. After that point, I continued to see a variety of parasites in my stool. I planned on continuing this cleanse for as long as it would take to rid myself of the creatures that were depleting my body of the important nutrients it needed to heal.

Parasites are not a pretty topic, but they're certainly worth addressing for the sake of your health. I will admit that I was originally apprehensive about starting this cleanse after hearing descriptions of the process and seeing pictures of what may come out of my body. I thought that once I saw what was inside of me, I would be so freaked out that I would cringe being in my own skin. However, once I saw evidence of the first parasite, I started to view it as a science experiment. I found myself researching the strange things coming out of me and thinking, "better out than in!"

In addition to the CellCore protocol, I continued to support my body's detox process by:
- Drinking plenty of clean, filtered water each day
- Spending time in my infrared sauna

- Partaking in coffee enemas every other day

The parasite cleanse ingredients can be mildly dehydrating, so the extra water intake, as well as the coffee enemas, helps your body release the toxins and parasites.

I was curious to see if the parasite cleanse would help me eliminate the toxic heavy metals in my body. I also was eager to find out if ridding myself of both the heavy metals and the parasites would relieve my remaining symptoms:

1. Brain fog and memory issues
2. Eczema in my ears
3. Nutritional deficiencies
4. Dark circles under my eyes

By this point, my stomach was extremely bloated, which I believed to be a side effect of the parasite cleanse. I began incorporating colonics into my routine once or twice a month to hydrate my colon and support the cleansing process. You can find a lot of literature about the benefits and cautions of colonics, so I won't go into it here. I'll just say that my personal research pointed to colonics as a powerful way to aid the parasite cleanse, decrease inflammation in my body, and boost my immune system.

To cover my bases, I decided to double-check that I didn't have Lyme or any associated infections, like Bartonella or Babesia. I had blood drawn and sent to the IGeneX Lab for testing in Palo Alto, California. When you're not getting 100% better, you must keep looking for the reason why. Bartonella is considered "the new Lyme" because it's transmitted in a similar fashion, but keep in mind that you can still have it without having Lyme. It's no longer considered a co-infection of Lyme, but rather an infection all on its own.

CHAPTER 35

Major Improvements

As March began to wind down, I found that my stomach was still noticeably bloated. I was unable to have a bowel movement, despite the fact that I religiously took a CALM magnesium supplement along with the "Bowel Mover" from CellCore. I suspected that something, such as a parasite, might have been blocking my intestines. I got into my infrared sauna for a session and then drank a few glasses of water. After that, I was finally able to go to the bathroom. I then did a coffee enema and went to my scheduled colonic appointment.

Goodbye, Gut Invaders!

About halfway through my colonic, a large parasite passed through the glass tube. The technician noted that she had not seen such a sizeable parasite in her office before but that it was most likely more visible in the clear water that resulted from my aggressive cleansing. When I got home, I replenished any vitamins and minerals that may have been lost during the colonic with some probiotics and a dose of trace minerals. The next morning, my stomach was no longer bloated.

I told myself there and then that I would continue the parasite cleanse and the coffee enemas, as well as the colonics, until any remaining parasites had made their final exit. Once you see what's been trapped inside your body with your own eyes, it becomes difficult to discontinue the elimination process.

One day, around mid-March, my foot felt fantastic. I felt like I could probably even have put on roller skates and gone around the rink without any discomfort, which, if you remember, was a goal of mine.

*

Some of the healing avenues you choose to take may seem drastic to others, but this is your journey. Don't ever forget that. If you feel strongly that you need to try something just to rule out the possibility of it affecting your health, don't let anyone shame you out of it.

CHAPTER 36

Continued Healing & Cleansing

On March 29, I received my test results from the naturopath. These would show whether I had Lyme, Babesia, or Bartonella. The results appeared to be negative for Babesia and Bartonella but were inconclusive for Borrelia burgdorferi — one of the parasites that causes Lyme. I knew that I could always redo the test in a couple of months for a hopefully more conclusive result, so in the meantime, I continued to cleanse.

By mid-April, I began noticing that I hadn't had any recent sugar cravings as I had had in the past. Usually, right before dinner, I would crave chocolate. This realization came to me when I noticed some almond peanut butter cups in my pantry but wasn't tempted in the least to reach for them. There's a theory that certain parasites make you crave sugar, so my suddenly tamed sweet tooth seemed like a good indication that the parasite cleanse was working!

A Healing Heart

As you become more devoted to taking care of yourself, you'll find that you have more abundant love for those around you. It's true what they say: you can't pour from an empty cup. I noticed how much I had grown into this state of love and gratitude at my daughter's college graduation.

What a great weekend that was! Not only did I get to see my daughter's achievement as she walked across the stage to receive her diploma, but I also experienced my own sense of achievement: my ex-husband and I spending time together. The best part of it all was that we really enjoyed each other's company.

It was a great feeling to reach this new emotional place with my ex-husband, and I look back on this as yet another step in my healing journey.

Affirmations for a Healed Heart

It's important to heal those old ties that bind you to past pain and trauma. We tend to hold emotional trauma in the body, and this can manifest itself as illness. If you'd like to let go of past pain and heal your heart, you can try the following daily affirmations:

- I am healing my heart.
- I am enough and worthy of love.
- I release the heartache from my past and wish my past love well.
- This is a fresh start for me and for them.

Rounding a Corner

By the end of April, I was using the infrared sauna more, doing coffee enemas every other day, and planning my next colonic. My cleansing efforts seemed to be working quite well because, at my next colonic, I expelled a large amount of waste. Initially, the water was very clear, and a semi-transparent parasite made an appearance. A few other parasite-related elements came out as well, resembling sandy-looking substances at the bottom of the tube. The technician informed me that these substances were, in fact, heavy metals, which gave me renewed faith in the fact that the heavy metal detox was really working its magic. I also released a lot of toxins. I was reassured that the combination of parasitic and heavy metal cleansing had to be done in this fashion, which would explain why I hadn't seen the same results before combining my efforts.

Even though I had stuck to this routine of coffee enemas followed by colonics in the past, I had never released so many toxins before. It made me wonder if any of this was tied to the emotional release I had recently experienced at my daughter's graduation. This serves as a prime example of how your psyche is connected to your physical well-being. This was further proven by the dreams that continued to filter in and out of my subconscious mind as I slept. Shortly after my colonic, I had a dream that I was at an event with a gigantic cake covered in thick icing. The cake must have been about the size of a tiny home. Someone in the crowd tossed me up on top of the cake and, as I crawled around on it, I pondered whether I should have a bite because I knew it had gluten in it. I couldn't resist and dug my whole hand into it, grabbing several big bites. When I woke from the dream, I was so relieved that I had not actually succumbed to my weakness and jeopardized my health.

Intermittent Fasting

In May, I continued with the Foundational Protocol from CellCore. This would be my fourth month on the cleanse, and I continued to supplement it with infrared sauna sessions and coffee enemas every other day. I was then inspired to try intermittent fasting, which consists of restricting meals (of standard portions) to a short window of time each day.

This eating regimen can help reduce inflammation, decrease your blood pressure, heart rate, and cholesterol, and even aid in reducing insulin resistance for people with diabetes. When you're digesting food, your body enters what is known as the "fed state," which lasts for about three to five hours from the moment you begin eating. In this state, your insulin levels are high, which makes it increasingly difficult to burn fat. Once your body reaches the post-absorptive state, which lasts for about 10 to 12 hours after your last meal, it's no longer absorbing any food. Following this timeframe is the fasted state. Because your insulin levels are low once again, this state allows your body to burn any dormant fat from the fed state.

While intermittent fasting can help you burn fat and reduce toxins, it's important to remember that this regimen doesn't give you free reign to eat unhealthy foods or the specific foods that your body is reactive to.

I found that I surprisingly didn't really miss food during the hours I spent fasting. I still had energy, and my stomach didn't feel overly full as it had in the past after eating my breakfast.

Exercise: Intermittent Fasting

Consult with your doctor before starting any fasting protocol to see if there are any contraindications for you personally. To start your intermittent fasting journey, I would recommend using the 16:8 ratio. This involves fasting for a 16-hour period and only eating within the allotted eight-hour window. You can follow the instructions below for a week and see how you feel:

1. Upon waking up, have a glass of warm water to dissolve any excess toxins in your digestive tract and get your bowels moving.
2. Follow this with a glass of cold water for better absorption and rehydration.
3. Try not to eat breakfast until 10 a.m.
4. Go about eating your normal meals throughout the day, with your last meal ending at 6 p.m.
5. Don't eat anything until 10 a.m. the following morning.
6. Repeat the process above for seven days.

If It Ain't Broke...

There's an old adage that says, "If it ain't broke, don't fix it." I fully believe that you should keep searching for newer, better ways to heal yourself completely, but that you should also do more of what's working for you. By the end of May, I started taking two capsules of S-acetyl glutathione each day, along with the other supplements that seemed to be working for me. S-acetyl glutathione has many known benefits, including its ability to fight free radicals and support detoxification. Its anti-inflammatory properties also assist in promoting brain and heart health. If you have issues with premature aging, dwindling energy, and low immunity, ask your practitioner about taking this supplement.

At this time, I was entering the sixth month of my CellCore Foundational Protocol. The positive effects of my routine were evidenced by:

- The release of parasites
- Decreased inflammation in my foot
- Noticeably thicker hair and stronger nails
- A curbed addiction to chocolate
- Enhanced mental focus

By July, I was ready for my phone consultation with Dr. Osborne, during which we went over the results of each test I had taken in the recent months.

Test	Result
MICRONUTRIENT TEST	I was deficient in several micronutrients, which meant I would need to take the recommended supplements for a two-month period.

Open-Minded Healing

My goal was to see, by September, if these deficiencies had been corrected. I would retake the test at that juncture. I would also continue to avoid gluten and other allergens in the meantime.

*

Test	Result
CARDIOMETABOLIC PANEL	These blood markers for assessing risk of metabolic syndrome and cardiovascular disease showed improvement from past results.

Overall, these tests showed a great deal of improvement in my health condition, for which I was encouraged and especially grateful. It's important to keep a log of all these tests. If you'd like to, you can use a format like the one below to track your progress. This will keep you motivated and give you better insight into what you need to be focusing your healing efforts on.

TEST	INITIAL RESULT	[DATE]	[DATE]	[DATE]
Write the specific test names.	Write the initial results of the corresponding test.	Write the results of the follow-up test.	Write the results of the follow-up test.	Write the results of the follow-up test.

Continue recording each subsequent test along with the date that the test was taken — not the date that the results were revealed. You may have made progress in the time between taking the test and going over the results, so this ensures more accurate recording.

CHAPTER 37

DENTISTRY WINS

It had now been three years and one month since my foot pain first surfaced. On October 23, I consulted with a biologic dentist to determine the best course of treatment for my infected root canal. The first step was to get a current X-ray of my root canal to better view the infected area. The scan showed the infection at the base of my root. The dentist informed me that the next step would be to remove the infected tooth and thoroughly clean out the surrounding tissue using different techniques as needed. I would quite possibly need ozone therapy to speed healing. To prepare my body and immune system for this procedure, the dentist suggested taking daily doses of <u>GMO-Free, Ultra Fine Vitamin C</u>, as well as <u>Non-GMO Chlorella Broken Cell Wall</u> capsules. I was asked to do this protocol at least two weeks prior to the surgery.

Once the procedure was completed, I would wait three months to ensure that no infection had set in. After that, I would have an implant placed in my jawbone. The dentist referred to my Biocompatibility Report and saw that my body seemed to be compatible with both titanium and ceramic implants.

NOTE: Some people, particularly those with autoimmune conditions, may have an adverse reaction to titanium.

Once the dental implant was securely in place, I would then have the ceramic tooth placed over it.

CHAPTER 38

The Future of Self-Healing

November saw me continuing with my parasite and heavy metal cleanse. I was encouraged by the progress that I was making, and I didn't want to stop the process too quickly. In my mind, this might have allowed the parasites to recolonize my digestive tract and deposit more heavy metals. There was no way I was letting that happen after how far I had come! The results of my health regimen were as follows:

- Hair continued to thicken
- Nails remained strong
- Complexion looked more youthful
- Chocolate cravings diminished significantly
- Bowel movements became more regular
- Nutrients seemed to be more readily absorbed; iron retention was normal for the first time in several years
- Rising at 6 a.m. wasn't an issue; feeling refreshed in the morning and going to bed by 10 p.m.

In addition to the CellCore protocol, I continued taking 100% pure organic chlorophyll tablets daily to support my heavy metal cleanse. I also purchased a personal FasciaBlaster: a product designed to help the body's connective tissue (known as fascia) detox and eliminate cellulite by breaking up fascial adhesions. It supposedly helped the creator, Ashley Black, heal her rheumatoid arthritis. I had heard so many positive reviews of this device, including a firsthand account from a friend, so I began using the FasciaBlaster on my legs and stomach alongside my dry brush before I showered.

I continued to do everything that I could to eliminate the damaging parasites and heavy metals from my body by supporting lymph, kidney, and liver drainage. (See The "How To" Handbook section under Resources on pgs. 171 & 172)

If there's one thing that you need to be aware of as you embark on your own healing journey, it's that improved health is not just a limited protocol you take on. It is a lifestyle that continues throughout your whole life. I continue to work on my health daily. I don't look at this as something I **have** to do, but rather as something I **want** to do. I choose to live in a state of inspiration as opposed to resistance.

All the steps I continue to take make me feel so much better and help me live life on my own terms — a life of freedom to do all the activities I want to do. I am now filled with an endless sense of excitement to live the life I want to lead.

CHAPTER 39

LOOKING BACK

"The most important things in life are the connections you make with others."

~Tom Ford

If you're not able to call on your family for any number of reasons, or if it doesn't feel like you're connected to a close group of friends, it's still possible to surround yourself with loving support. If you make it a point to be open and allow yourself to be vulnerable — and accept help from others — you will encourage a flow of good deeds on your behalf.

Prior to my diagnosis, I had been feeling very apathetic and alone. Autoimmune conditions, overall, often fuel feelings of depression or anxiety. This is not only because of your body's inability to absorb important nutrients and balance hormones but because of feelings of isolation and fear of what the future might hold. The silver lining of this illness was that it brought so much love, kindness, and connection into my life!

Soon after my diagnosis, I remember asking myself what the lesson was that I was supposed to learn. Maybe it was accepting help from others. I told myself that I would accept help from the next person who offered it since I wanted to get past this lesson quickly.

After allowing myself to accept help from the first person who offered, the good deeds multiplied exponentially. A key turning point was the moment I hobbled on my crutches past a grocery store on my way to the coffee shop. After getting my typical green tea latte with coconut milk, I awkwardly headed to the exit, trying not to spill the drink while navigating my way around on crutches. Before I had even reached the door, I saw a young man standing there, patiently waiting to open it for me. He said that he had been in the grocery store when I passed by the window earlier and thought I might like some help shopping. A man who had been nothing more than a complete stranger moments before had gone out of his way to find me and ask if I needed assistance.

In the past, the independent me would have told him his assistance wasn't necessary. However, the new me — the person who wanted to learn their lesson quickly — accepted his assistance with gratitude, despite the fact that I wasn't originally planning on stocking up on groceries that day. He patiently waited for me as we made our way through the store, picking up items I pointed out and placing them in his shopping cart as we continued to chat. I found out that when he was in college, he had broken his neck and needed to wear special headgear to stabilize it for many months. He still remembered how difficult the experience had been, which is why he had felt so compelled to reach out to help me.

Anyone who has been on crutches for any length of time can relate to how difficult it is to get around on them. It was so exhausting that when I wasn't able to find a close enough parking space, I would simply admit defeat and drive away from the shopping center without ever getting out of the car. Once I received my handicap sign in the mail, it made it easier to park closer to the store whenever there were handicap spots available.

NOTE: For those of you who have reduced mobility due to your condition, you can fill out an application for a handicap sign through your local DMV.

Initially, the crutches took getting used to, and I remember some major falls, including one where I lost my balance and ended up injuring my good foot to avoid falling on the injured one. I am very independent and would often take on more than I should have while on crutches, like trying to get around the grocery store while carrying my groceries in a bag. One day, the grocery store manager saw me and came running over with a horrified expression, insisting that I wait while he got me a motorized chair. He may have been thinking about how good it felt to help someone — as well as to avoid a potential lawsuit!

Perhaps that is the greatest lesson of all. Hardship is not meant to make us harder, but rather softer in our approaches to those around us. It's meant to open our eyes and reconnect us to the loving feeling that we should be giving and receiving on a daily basis.

Looking back, I wish I could have acknowledged every act of kindness that I received and every person who offered it, but there are too many to even recall. I expected the world to be kind, and it listened.

Paying it Forward

Doing nice things for others can have such a profound impact on your life. Whether you become part of a group that helps other people or just make it a point to be nice to everyone you run into throughout the day, always try to pay kindness forward. You can find a group to work with through your church, a food pantry, or a volunteer organization. If you're going to be making it a point to be nicer, look people in the eye and say hello, share genuine compliments out loud, give someone a great Yelp review, or offer your server a generous tip. Even if you're wheelchair-bound, confined by crutches, or strained financially, there are so many ways to spread kindness that don't cost a single cent. When you extend kindness to yourself and others while expecting the world around you to be kind, you will see it reflected back to you.

While it can take a conscious effort to exude positivity, exercising this muscle becomes easier with time and can be incredibly beneficial to your overall well-being.

Suggested Protocol for Healing

I do want to remind you that healing is a process, and I didn't tackle everything at the same time. I'm giving you all the information I acquired over the course of the two- to three-year period I spent searching for solutions. I don't want you to get overwhelmed by the specifics you're about to read. Instead, take it one day and one protocol at a time and have patience with the process (and, more importantly, yourself) along the way.

The first thing you'll need to do if you suspect that you have an autoimmune or autoinflammatory illness is remove all gluten, grains, dairy, soy, corn, peanuts, alcohol, nightshades, caffeine, and processed foods and sugars or artificial sweeteners from your diet. This will provide your body with a hard reset and allow it to heal without the inflammation that gluten, grains, and dairy have put it through. Corn is on the list because it's typically a genetically modified organism (GMO) that is high in lectins and hard to digest.

"For one, lectins tend to bind to fibers in your small intestine. As a result, you can't absorb the nutrients in your food properly. Secondly, lectins also attach to insulin receptors, making you more insulin resistant." (13)

Alcohol creates deficiencies in B vitamins and minerals, which our body needs for healing. Caffeine can make it difficult for our adrenal glands to recover and may contribute to low energy levels and the inability to exercise effectively. Nightshades, including lentils, legumes (especially peanuts), eggplants, peppers, and potatoes present a challenge to digestion as well. Eat organic as often as possible to avoid glyphosate (the weed-killing Roundup sprayed on crops).

A great resource is Dr. Peter Osborne's book, *No Grain, No Pain*. Dr. Osborne also offers a wealth of free information about autoimmune recovery, as well as a range of delicious recipes, on glutenfreesociety.org. You can find a link to his book in the Recommended Reading & Listening section at the end of this book.

You can also check out Dr. Josh Axe's program online. He is a certified doctor of natural medicine, clinical nutritionist, and Doctor of Chiropractic who focuses on the art of ancient medicine. There are a few paid programs that he offers, and you can pick one that's related to your personal health conditions. You'll get access to recipes, support, and a private Facebook group — well worth the investment if you ask me.

Next, you'll need to find yourself a knowledgeable naturopath or functional medicine doctor to help you navigate your return to a balanced state of health. I wouldn't suggest going it alone without the support of someone whose expertise has helped many others heal. Whoever you settle on will need to be able to run you through the necessary tests to determine what's really going on in your body. The main tests that I've found very helpful, as well as tests your doctor may recommend, include:

1. Vitamin and Mineral Deficiency Panel
2. Heavy Metal Test
3. Iron and Vitamin D Level Testing

4. Food Allergy Testing, plus a Delayed Sensitivity Test
5. Stool Test (checks for parasites, inflammation markers, bacteria overgrowth such as H. pylori, and much more)
6. Cardiometabolic Testing
7. Neurotransmitter Test (confirms levels of serotonin, GABA, dopamine, noradrenaline, adrenaline, and glutamate)

After this, you'll need to address parasitic overload, even if parasites don't show up in your stool test. Many people have parasites and simply aren't aware of it. I personally used the Foundational Protocol from CellCore and was visually able to see, within a short amount of time, that I had parasites.

Next up on your agenda, you'll need to address heavy metals in your system. We're all bombarded by these heavy metals on a regular basis and need to detox them correctly. Your practitioner can help guide you properly through this process. Dr. Klinghardt also offers many free online videos that address proper detoxification protocols for heavy metals that you may find helpful.

Lastly, I want to emphasize the importance of STRESS and the negative role it plays on your health. Find healthy ways to mitigate stress in your life or address any trauma you've experienced. Some therapeutic methods you may find effective for releasing trauma are Eye Movement Desensitization and Reprocessing (EMDR) therapy, Somatic Breathwork, Emotional Freedom Technique (EFT) tapping, and the Fascial Counterstrain work created by Brian Tuckey to help a vast number of conditions, including PTSD.

Other Areas to Focus On:
1. Check for mold in your home.
2. Develop a strong support system of friends, family, and doctors.

3. Focus on daily meditation. It's a great stress reliever that will positively affect your health. It will also help make you aware of solutions that you may not have thought of previously.
4. Use a Far Infrared heating pad or find a place where you can use a Far Infrared sauna. Both options help with detoxification, inflammation, and sleep. IV therapy can also assist in bolstering your immune system and aiding the detoxification process.
5. Consider working with a certified acupuncturist. It is amazing how beneficial acupuncture can be for your health.

Finally, do the things that make you happy! This is something you hear all the time but, surprisingly, many people don't prioritize this for a variety of reasons. Some people think that it's too self-indulgent, or they feel guilty for doing something that is just for themselves. Some people become addicted to their negative emotions. Others haven't taken the time to figure out what actually makes them happy or just don't realize the positive impact it will have on their own health and well-being. One thing to note is that prioritizing your happiness won't just have a positive impact on you but on those that love and depend on you as well.

I would suggest giving yourself a gift each week, either as a reward for the steps you took to better your health or simply as a way to put yourself in a state of appreciation and joy. You could treat yourself to a foot soak with Epsom and lavender salts, buy a beautiful bouquet of flowers at your next trip to the grocery store, write yourself a note expressing gratitude for your positive traits, or immerse yourself in nature by taking a walk somewhere new.

CHAPTER 40

Parting Advice

I want to emphasize how important it is to do your own research and be vocal in your doctor's office. I became my own best advocate from the very beginning of this journey because I knew that speaking up for myself was the only way to get this disease under control.

I saw a variety of doctors, never relying solely on the opinion of one. Instead, I took in information from the medical professionals and did all my own online research. I chose to listen to my own body and intuition about what I would implement and what simply didn't work. I started my office visits off by telling each doctor that I was only interested in solutions. I didn't need all their dire outlooks or worst-case scenarios milling around in my head, nor did I want my subconscious to start conjuring the symptoms that I had just heard about. The doctors may have written some interesting things about me in their notes, but I truly didn't care. My only priority was taking care of myself to the best of my ability.

In my opinion, there are many reasons why people aren't healing from these autoimmune conditions.

Why Aren't People Healing?

1. Some believe that the MDs are the only authority on the matter and choose to ignore all other healing modalities because of this line of thinking.

2. Others prefer the seemingly easier measure of taking medications over making major lifestyle changes.
3. Some are too overwhelmed with all the information. This makes them feel like they don't know where to even begin, so they remain stuck.
4. Some are too addicted to the various substances they rely on to help pull them out of pain or depression. This could include nicotine, sugary treats, pain pills, and much more. This addiction makes it too difficult to take on the daunting task of letting go of certain vices to overcome all these health obstacles.
5. Some may lack the emotional support at home that they need to follow through with the hard work of healing.
6. Some are too depressed because of the disease itself and lack the necessary daily guidance to get through this difficult transition.
7. Some start a healing protocol but give up too soon before they can start seeing the benefits.
8. Some have lived so long with their condition that they are immune to just how badly they feel, not realizing that feeling better is an option.
9. Some don't believe anything could make them feel better.
10. Others don't want to even dare to hope for a healthier life only to be drastically disappointed with the outcome.

Believe me, I know it takes hard work to change your lifestyle completely! I do believe that the first month is the hardest of them all. This is a time when you'll be releasing sugar, dairy, and gluten-laden grains from your diet. You'll be challenging your body in various other ways on both an emotional and physical level. However, once you start seeing the results of your new lifestyle and the impact that it has on your well-being, you'll be inspired and encouraged to continue this new way of life. You'll also find solace in the fact that it is leading you on a journey where the final destination is optimal health!

If you can overcome those challenges — those reasons why most people don't heal — you'll have a far better outlook.

Find Your Why

Another piece of my parting advice is to find your "why." Walking this journey requires commitment. I was very determined to take difficult measures and drastically change my lifestyle because I couldn't bear the idea of being in pain for the rest of my life. I would do anything to avoid it. When you begin trying to establish your "why," I want you to ask yourself a few questions:

- What is the reason you would stay on this path?
- Is it because you want to be around later for your children and grandchildren?
- Is it because you want to show strength amidst adversity and take this as a challenge?
- Is it because you desperately want to get back to work or some semblance of normal daily functioning without constant pain and depression?
- Is it because you've gotten to the point of "all or nothing" and don't want to continue life in a way that's just too physically and emotionally painful?

It's extremely important to have a compelling "why" that will continually motivate you throughout every step of your healing journey. It's just as important as having hope that a brighter future lies ahead.

If you'd like to keep in touch or be informed about upcoming events or the latest Open-Minded Healing podcast episodes, visit openmindedhealing.com.

Thank you for reading this book. My hope is that it has provided you with information and inspiration that leads to less pain, more love and connection, and the healthy future you envision for yourself.

Wishing you all optimal health,

Marla Miller

RESOURCES

The "How To" Handbook

1. Ways to Support Lymphatic Drainage:
- Sleep with the head of the bed raised by 5 inches. (You can purchase a "wedge" online or put blocks under the feet of the head of your bed.)
- Jump on a mini trampoline each day.
- Dry brush your body.
- Use the FasciaBlaster to break up fascia and increase circulation.
- Sleep between the hours of 10 p.m. and 6 a.m. This is the time period when your brain actually shrinks to allow for lymph drainage, according to Dr. Klinghardt.
- Perform lymph massages. You can try some of Dr. Klinghardt's techniques on his YouTube channel.

2. Ways to Support Kidney and Liver Drainage:
- Drink a glass of water with lemon first thing in the morning to help cleanse toxins from your system.
- Drink herbal teas, such as dandelion or nettle tea.
- Drink plenty of purified water throughout the day.
- Avoid foods or beverages that put a strain on the kidneys while doing a cleanse. These foods include:
  - Caffeine
  - Alcohol

- Nuts
- Foods that are refined or harder for the kidneys to process, such as fats and proteins

3. Meditation

By making meditation a daily habit, you can rely on it an effective tool for downloading solutions from your higher consciousness. It will also begin to affect you on a physiological, biological, and emotional level. For more information on how meditation impacts your health, feel free to dive into Dr. Joe Dispenza's scientific research.

Before You Get Started:
- Make a commitment to your meditation practice. Start by telling yourself that you will only be doing this for 10 minutes a day. Engage in meditations around the same time each day to establish a solid routine. Try to meditate when you're least distracted by external sources. I gradually increased my meditation time until I found that sweet spot where there was enough time for me to immerse myself in the experience and reach the point of blocking out everything around me. On a physical level, I would compare this state to the times when your body matches the temperature of bathwater so perfectly that you're no longer aware of the water touching your skin. When I get deep enough into meditation, I cannot feel my own body sitting on the couch. Personally, I find that 30 minutes of meditation works well, but you may find you can reach that space in just 10 minutes.
- Decide if you prefer meditating with music, a guided meditation, or in silence. One of my personal favorites, when I want music on, is one of Deva Premal's many meditation songs. Her voice

lulls me into the perfect state of mind for being present in the moment and helps me to release any distractions. When I'm in the mood for a guided meditation, I enjoy <u>Getting Into the Vortex</u> by Abraham, Esther, and Jerry Hicks. Wayne Dyer also has a guided meditation available, as well as Deepak Chopra and Oprah Winfrey, who offer 21-day guided meditations. Depending on the meditation in question, you may be able to find one for free or for purchase. If you prefer silence, you can start by asking yourself questions internally, such as:

- Who am I?
- What is my purpose?
- What do I really, really want?

Doing so helps provide the space to focus on your intentions and listen for the answers the Universe provides. However, it's not necessary to ask any questions at all. You may just want to sit in silence and enjoy the benefits of turning the chatter of your brain off.

Time to Meditate:
- Find a comfortable, peaceful spot to meditate where you won't be disrupted. (It can be helpful to create a clean, decluttered space for this purpose. You can even add a candle, a little Buddha statue, or anything that symbolizes tranquility to you. I personally like to sage the whole house before I sink into meditation.)
- Sit down and get comfortable with both feet flat on the floor and your hands in your lap.
- Take two or three deep breaths, inhaling through your nose and exhaling out through your mouth slowly. I usually draw a deep breath in for a count of five seconds, hold the breath for a count of five seconds, and then release the breath for a count of 10 seconds.

NOTE: Initially, when you begin this practice, it's very common to be distracted by all of your thoughts. That's completely normal! If you fall asleep easily, it probably means you need more sleep or should be picking a different time of day to meditate. You want to be completely relaxed, but not so relaxed that you'll fall soundly asleep. It should feel more like you just lost track of time. The more you try not to think, the more distracted you'll be. It's important to allow space for whatever thoughts come up. Just notice what you're thinking and then bring your focus back to your breath or to a mantra.

Example Mantras:
- I am enough.
- I am healing.
- I am getting stronger and calmer.
- I am loved and I embody love.
- I am open to the possibilities that the Universe has in store for me.
- I am filled with gratitude.
- I am whole.
- I am worthy.
- I am at peace.
- I feel my health being restored.

4. Coffee Enemas

You will need:

An enema bucket and tube (I prefer the metal version over the plastic one)
- Organic coconut oil or another organic lubricant
- A non-aluminum pot or saucepan
- A strainer

- 4 cups of filtered or distilled water
- 3 rounded tbsp. of finely ground organic coffee — not instant (I used S.A. Wilson's Gold Roast)
- A timer
- Any relaxing music you might like to listen to during the process

To Get Started:
- Measure out 4 cups of purified or filtered water and put it in a saucepan. Add 2-3 tbsp. of organic coffee.
- Bring the water and coffee to a boil, then reduce the heat to a medium temperature, allowing it to slowly boil for 3 minutes.
- After 3 minutes, turn the burner to the lowest setting and let it simmer for 12 minutes.
- Turn the burner off and strain the coffee grinds using a small strainer, pouring the coffee into a separate container.
- Allow the mixture to cool down.
- Once the coffee has cooled down to a tepid temperature (where it doesn't feel hot or cold), it is ready.
- Put some coconut oil in a small container.
- Place a towel on the bathroom floor, along with the container of coconut oil and your timer.
- Pour the coffee into the bucket with the tubing attached.
- Make sure the valve is closed when doing this!
- Hang the bucket about 16 inches above the place where you'll be lying down.
- Lubricate the tubing with the coconut oil before inserting it into your rectum.
- Set your timer to 15 minutes.

- Release about 2 cups of the coffee mixture at a time. (Essentially, this means you'll be doing two enemas, 2 cups at a time.)
- Leave it in place for 15 minutes to reap the full benefits of the enema.
- Cautiously stand up, get to the toilet, sit down, and release the coffee from your system.
- Once you've completely evacuated your bowels, lie back down and repeat the process with the final 2 cups.

TOP TIP: Clean the bucket and tubing out with warm, soapy water, then drain them completely before hanging them up to dry thoroughly.

5. Parasitic Cleansing

To cleanse your body of any parasites, I would recommend ordering a CellCore Foundational Protocol Kit through your naturopath or functional medicine practitioner.

6. Autoimmune Conditions & Their Symptoms

Addison's disease	• Exhaustion • Weight loss • Dizziness when standing • Low blood pressure • Muscle weakness • Frequent urination • Depression • Darkened patches of skin
Celiac disease	• Constipation • Bloating • Lactose intolerance • Loose, greasy stools • Abdominal pain • Nausea and/or vomiting

Dermatomyositis	- Red or purple rash on sun-exposed skin - Muscle weakness - Trouble talking - Trouble swallowing
Grave's disease	- Anxiety - Irritability - Hand tremors - Weight loss - Thyroid goiter - Menstrual cycle changes
Hashimoto's thyroiditis	- Fatigue - Unexplained weight gain - Intolerance to cold - Constipation - Joint & muscle aches - Slow heart rate - Heavy menstrual cycles - Dry skin - Thin hair
Multiple sclerosis	- Muscle stiffness and spasms - Blurry vision - Bladder control issues - Numbness or tingling in the body - Poor coordination & balance - Fatigue - Difficulty walking
Myasthenia gravis	- Droopy eyelids - Trouble making facial expressions - Slurred speech - Double vision - Weak arms and legs - Shortness of breath - Trouble chewing & swallowing

Pernicious anemia	- Fatigue - Confusion - Impaired sense of smell - Numbness in hands and/or feet - Jaundice - Rapid heart rate
Reactive arthritis	- Inflammation of the eyes - Urinary tract issues - Swollen toes and/or fingers - Lower back pain - Pain & stiffness in joints - Tendon inflammation
Rheumatoid arthritis	- Aches & pains in multiple joints - Stiffness in more than one joint - Weight loss - Fever - Fatigue - Weakness - Tenderness & swelling of the joints
Sjogren's syndrome	- Dry eyes - Dry skin - Dry mouth - Vaginal dryness - Tiredness - Muscular & joint pain - Swollen salivary glands - Rash
Systemic lupus erythematosus	- Fatigue - Malaise - Loss of appetite - Fever - Joint pain - Skin issues - Muscular pain & weakness

Type I diabetes	• Extreme thirst
	• Urinary frequency
	• Weight loss
	• Thrush
	• Slow healing cuts, grazes, and bruises
	• Blurry vision
	• Fatigue
	• Fruity breath
Ankylosing spondylitis	• Morning stiffness
	• Pain and stiffness in the lower back and/or hips
	• Neck pain
	• Fatigue
	• Joint stiffness
	• Joint inflammation
	• Inflammation of the middle layer of the eye

While the list of symptoms under each condition is not exhaustive, this will give you a good idea of what you might be dealing with.

Recommended Reading & Listening

For Diet:

Osborne, Peter, PhD. (2016). **No Grain, No Pain: A 30-Day Diet for Eliminating the Root Cause of Chronic Pain**. Atria Paperback. New York.

Dr. Josh Axe's Ancient Medicine Programs. https://draxe.com/program-login/

For Inspiration:

Moorjani, Anita. (2012). **Dying To Be Me: My Journey from Cancer, to Near Death, to True Healing**. Hay House. New York.

Dyer, Wayne, D.C. **Divine Love** audiobook.

Dispenza, Joe. (2013). **Breaking the Habit of Being Yourself: How to Lose Your Mind and Create a New One.**

For Meditating:

Esther Hicks (Author), Jerry Hicks (Author). (2010). **Getting Into the Vortex: Guided Meditations CD and User Guide"**

Deva Premal meditation music. https://www.youtube.com/watch?v=yQjHSIHPJfw

Wholetones: Music for Peace, Healing, Sleep, and Energy. https://wholetones.com/

Source — It's Within You documentary. https://sourcethefilm.org/home/

For Clearing Clutter:

Kingston, Karen. (2016). **Clear Your Clutter With Feng Shui.** Harmony Books.

Kondo, Marie. (2014). **The Life-Changing Magic of Tidying Up: The Japanese Art of Decluttering and Organizing**. Berkeley: Ten Speed Press.

For Rheumatoid Arthritis:

Scammell, Henry & McPherson Brown, Thomas. (2016). **The Road Back: Rheumatoid Arthritis — Its Cause and Its Treatment.**

References & Citations

Stoltzfus, Seth. Medically reviewed by Murrell, Daniel, M.D. (2018). *Addisonian Crisis (Acute Adrenal Crisis)*. Healthline.

Scammell, Henry & McPherson Brown, Thomas. (2016). *The Road Back: Rheumatoid Arthritis — Its Cause and Its Treatment*. Rowman & Littlefield Publishers. London.

Nayaswami Jyotish, Nayaswami Devi. (2014). *The Tremendous Power of Meditation.* Ananda. https://www.ananda.org/jyotish-and-devi/tremendous-power-meditation/

Scammell, Henry & McPherson Brown, Thomas. (2016). *The Road Back: Rheumatoid Arthritis — Its Cause and Its Treatment*. Rowman & Littlefield Publishers. London.

Greger, Michael, M.D. (2017). *Plant vs. Animal Iron.* NutritionFacts.org. https://nutritionfacts.org/blog/plant-versus-animal-iron/

Singer, Michael. (2007). *The Untethered Soul: The Journey Beyond Yourself.* New Harbinger Publications.

Singer, Michael. (2007). *The Untethered Soul: The Journey Beyond Yourself.* New Harbinger Publications.

Abu-Shakra, M., & Shoenfeld, Y. (1991). *Parasitic infection and autoimmunity.* Autoimmunity. https://doi.org/10.3109/08916939108997136

Moorjani, Anita. (2012). *Dying to Be Me: My Journey from Cancer, to Near Death, to True Healing.* Hay House. New York.

Ortner, Nick. (2013). *The Tapping Solution: A Revolutionary System for Stress-Free Living.* Hay House.

Myers, Amy, M.D. (2024). *The MTHFR Mutation: What It Is and What To Do About It.* Amy Myers M.D. https://www.amymyersmd.com/blogs/articles/mthfr-mutation

Son, H., Song, H. J., Seo, H. J., Lee, H., Choi, S. M., & Lee, S. (2020). *The safety and effectiveness of self-administered coffee enema: A systematic review of case reports.* Medicine, 99(36), e21998. https://doi.org/10.1097/MD.0000000000021998

Virgin, JJ. (2023). *Why corn might be more harmful than you think.* JJ Virgin. https://jjvirgin.com/quick-question-whats-wrong-corn/

www.ingramcontent.com/pod-product-compliance
Lightning Source LLC
Chambersburg PA
CBHW020541030426
42337CB00013B/936